FOR TOTAL STRENGTH, PEACE OF MIND, AND OVERALL WELL-BEING . . . HERE ARE JUST A FEW SIMPLE AND DELICIOUS RECIPES TO REVITALIZE YOUR BODY'S BONE REGENERATION POTENTIAL

- **Salmon Omelet with Fresh D**
  An elegant dish for brunch or

- **Cajun Kale**
  A zesty Louisiana side dish

- **Cilantro–Egg Drop Soup**
  Perfect for a light spring lunch

- **Gingered Vegetable Caviar with Tofu and Dried Mushrooms**
  A sensational side dish served hot or cold

- **Chick Pea Tabouli**
  A tasty appetizer for parties, picnics, and snacks

ANNEMARIE COLBIN, a food therapist and leading expert on natural food and healing has an M.A. in Holistic Nutrition and is a Certified Health Education Specialist (C.H.E.S.). She is the founder of the Natural Gourmet Cookery School and Institute for Food and Health in New York, where she teaches regularly. Her work has been featured in the *New York Times, Elle, Good Housekeeping, Natural Health, Longevity,* and *New Age Journal* and she has been a columnist of *Free Spirit* since 1988. She has appeared on numerous talk shows, including "Live with Regis and Kathy Lee," "Donahue," and the TV Food Network and is the winner of a National IACP/Seagram Book Award for *The Natural Gourmet* and the 1993 Avon Women of Enterprise Award. Ms. Colbin lives in New York City with her husband, journalist Bernard Gavzer.

FOOD
and
OUR BONES

The Natural Way to Prevent Osteoporosis

Annemarie Colbin, M.A., C.H.E.S.

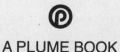

A PLUME BOOK

A NOTE TO THE READER
The ideas, procedures, and suggestions contained in this book are not intended as a substitute for medical treatment by a physician. The reader should regularly consult a physician in matters relating to health.

PLUME
Published by the Penguin Group
Penguin Putnam Inc., 375 Hudson Street, New York, New York 10014, U.S.A.
Penguin Books Ltd, 27 Wrights Lane, London W8 5TZ, England
Penguin Books Australia Ltd, Ringwood, Victoria, Australia
Penguin Books Canada Ltd, 10 Alcorn Avenue, Toronto, Ontario, Canada M4V 3B2
Penguin Books (N.Z.) Ltd, 182–190 Wairau Road, Auckland 10, New Zealand

Penguin Books Ltd, Registered Offices: Harmondsworth, Middlesex, England

First published by Plume, an imprint of Dutton NAL, a member of Penguin Putnam Inc.

First Printing, July, 1998

10   9   8   7   6   5

LIBRARY OF CONGRESS CATALOGING-IN-PUBLICATION DATA:

Colbin, Annemarie.
    Food and our bones : the natural way to prevent osteoporosis / Annemarie Colbin.
    p.   cm.
    Includes bibliographical references and index.
    ISBN 0-452-27806-6
    1. Osteoporosis—Popular works. 2. Osteoporosis—Prevention. 3. Osteoporosis—Diet therapy.
I. Title.
RC931.073C64   1998
616.16—dc21   97-53118
                                                                                    CIP

Printed in the United States of America
Set in Adobe Garamond
Designed by Eve L. Kirch

BOOKS ARE AVAILABLE AT QUANTITY DISCOUNTS WHEN USED TO PROMOTE PRODUCTS OR SERVICES. FOR INFORMATION PLEASE WRITE TO PREMIUM MARKETING DIVISION, PENGUIN PUTNAM INC., 375 HUDSON STREET, NEW YORK, NEW YORK 10014.

Dedicated with love to all my friends who worry about their bones, and to my husband, Bernie Gavzer, who doesn't worry about anything.

ACKNOWLEDGMENTS

My thanks first of all to publisher Elaine Koster of Dutton Signet, who approached me with the idea of writing about this subject. Without her steady encouragement, I would probably not have dared tackle it. Editor Deirdre Mullane went through the manuscript in what I consider record speed, and always had valuable feedback and suggestions. My agent and friend, Sarah Jane Freymann, rescued me several times from writer's stumbles, kept me on purpose, and was invariably on target with her advice.

Thanks go to Darwin Marcus Johnson, a graduate of The Natural Gourmet Cookery School, for his expert help with recipe testing and his good suggestions, and to Helen Lyu for all the research material she found for me. Also to Kelly Annotti at ESHA Research for providing me with extra nutritional data, and to Lisa Oehrl at Southern Research and Testing for attending to the nutritional testing of several of my recipes. Mark Liponis, M.D., a physician at Canyon Ranch in the Berkshires, was kind enough to provide me with further research and his medical comments on the manuscript. My friend Christiane Northrup, M.D., opened my mind with her always penetrating insights into the nature of being female. Nina Merer generously shared her personal experience in strengthening her bones the natural way. Thomas Cowan, M.D., and Sally Fallon provided me with valuable information.

Thanks to my husband Bernie and to all our children for being who they are, my most important support system. Most of all, my thanks to the spirits of my mother, Johanna Cornelia Polonyi-Stridiron, and my aunt, Geertruida Stridiron-Van Osch, who provided me with good role models to follow.

CONTENTS

FOREWORD

Few medical conditions epitomize the importance of balance as completely as osteoporosis. This balancing act involves a complex interplay between nutrition, genetics, and lifestyle. The effects of this interplay can be seen on many levels—biochemical, cellular, individual, and societal.

Optimal bone density is a reflection of one's overall health. Imbalances caused by alterations in nutrition, activity level, mood or mental state, medications, alcohol or other substances, or a disease process all have an effect on bone density. Optimal bone density requires *balance*.

On a biochemical level, the balance of hormones including the thyroid, parathyroid, adrenal, gonadal, and growth hormones interact with Vitamin D, calcium, phosphate, and a host of local regulators and growth factors to continuously modulate bone structure and strength. Each of these, either in deficiency or in excess, have been associated with disorders of bone. The complex interplay among these hormones are a reflection of each individual's overall health and stage in life. The skeleton advances along its own "life cycle"; immature bone matrix in childhood, mineralization during adolescence, maturation during early adulthood leading to peak bone mass, maintenance throughout middle age, rapid bone turnover associated with menopause, and the slow bone loss of aging. Each stage is affected by one's overall health, hormones, and nutrition.

On a cellular level, "bone remodeling units" comprised of osteoblast and osteoclast cells support the continuous cycle of forming new bone and reabsorbing old bone. The activity and balance of this system is controlled by many factors including nutrition, hormones, exercise, as well as gravitational, physical, and emotional stress. Imbalance of any of these factors can favor osteoclast cells which reabsorb bone, leading to progressively weaker bones and ultimately osteoporosis. Conversely, factors which enhance osteoblast activity lead to increased deposition of new bone and progressively denser bones. The long term balance of this microscopic system of "bone remodeling units" ultimately determines overall bone mineral content and bone density.

On a societal level, the incidence of osteoporosis is increasing at alarming rates. Current estimates place the financial burden of the disorder at $10 billion annually, with a projected $45.2 billion expected just ten years from now. Forces contributing to this increased burden include a growing aged population, a trend toward more sedentary occupations and less daily physical activity, the increasing reliance on motorized transportation, and an omnious deterioration of nutrition, particularly among adolescents and teens who are in the process of building their skeletons and achieving their peak bone mass by their early twenties. The increasing incidence of osteoporosis worldwide would seem to indicate a societal imbalance of sorts. Balancing societal forces which optimistically will limit the explosive incidence of osteoporosis include recent scientific developments in the understanding of the disorder itself; improvements in the accuracy, availability, and cost of screening; advances in treatment and in preventive strategies; as well as an overall heightening of global health awareness and concerns. Of these positive forces, the most important is prevention.

Prevention of osteoporosis is an issue of balance. Current research suggests that it is not simply deficiencies which result in osteoporosis; excesses of many nutrients including calcium, protein, sodium, and even exercise have been shown to aggravate osteoporosis and skeletal deformities. More is not necessarily better. Excessive calcium and vitamin D supplementation have been associated with increased fracture rates. The importance of balanced nutrition should not be underestimated, and hence the value of sound nutritional advice.

Food and Our Bones offers just such sage advice. Annemarie Colbin has skillfully blended her intimate knowledge of food with a deep understanding of balance to produce this valuable book. This common sense approach provides an excellent basis for understanding the relationship between our bones and our diet.

Mark Liponis, M.D.
Medical Director, Canyon Ranch
Lenox, Massachusetts
January 1998

One farmer says to me, "You cannot live on vegetable food solely, for it furnishes nothing to make bones with"; and so he religiously devotes a part of his day to supplying his system with the raw material of bones; walking all the while he talks behind his oxen, which, with vegetable made bones, jerk him and his lumbering plow along in spite of every obstacle. Some things are really necessaries of life in some circles, the most helpless and diseased, which in others are luxuries merely, and in others still are entirely unknown.

Henry David Thoreau, *Walden*

INTRODUCTION

Like the rest of us, I'm getting older. However, I feel very strongly that getting older is a joyful process of growing and learning; it is neither illness nor mistake. Society, on the other hand, insists that for a woman it is both. We are bombarded with advice on how to "stay young," "gain eternal youth," "drop years from your appearance," often by taking various kinds of drugs and pills that will try to keep our bodies hormonally the same as they were for their thirty or forty reproductive years. We are told to "shape up," "lose weight," "banish wrinkles," get our faces lifted and our bodies liposucked.

I say, what for? At thirty, our sexual energy is at its peak. At sixty, our sexual energy can be at a steady and comfortable hum; at the same time, our spiritual energy is rising. Why hold on to the past and confuse the issue? At a time in history when there is enough food, shelter, safety from predators (well, it's either the lions or the muggers, and I think city life can be as safe as life in the jungle)—we can live long and productive lives, and really contribute our wisdom and experience to the world. Why should we pretend to be sweet young things when we are mature women?

Believe it or not, this brings me to the subject at hand. Among women around the menopause, the subject of osteoporosis and brittle bones is a major concern. Hardly a day goes by when I don't see it mentioned somewhere, or don't talk to a woman who is worried about it. More and more, osteoporosis looks like the subject of a major publicity campaign. However, it *is* true that broken hips, broken backs, and broken wrists occur frequently in older people in our society, so the issue warrants attention.

Bones are supposed to last a long time. There are fossil bones that have been lying around for hundreds of thousands of years! Why is it that over the past decade osteoporosis has become such an issue? It never has been before: when I checked into all the old health and nutrition books that I own, bones are hardly mentioned, and osteoporosis is not to be found in the indexes. Today, a few years away from the millennium, on the other hand, osteoporosis is a major public health concern, there are all kinds of books written about it, and millions of women are swallowing millions of pills to keep it at bay. What is it about our lives today that is having such a negative impact on our body's inner structure? Can this unnatural process be stopped or reversed by taking a few pills?

I have my doubts. Health issues are extremely complex. They comprise many details and variables that interact with and balance each other; usually, if one of them changes, the others change as well. In the social communication of health concepts, many variables are often reduced to just a few; these are then the ones that are presented as the only essential concepts, while the others are abandoned or ignored.

This is what has happened with the thinning of the bones that can indicate risk of fracture, most commonly in old age. Osteoporosis can occur from a number of causes, including nutrition, lifestyle factors, illness, and steroid drug use. However, news reports about the issue have reduced it to two main causes: lack of calcium and lack of estrogen. While the condition happens to men as well as to women, it has been the women who have been targeted by the marketing campaigns of those who sell drugs and milk products. Older, alcoholic men are at serious risk for osteoporosis and bone fractures as well; why aren't they also targeted for testosterone replacement therapy? What we are actually being sold is a large helping of fear, and we women all too often allow ourselves to be manipulated, scared, or even made to feel we are acting responsibly if we follow our fear. Because of that fear, women are swallowing calcium pills and estrogen pills by the ton, even if they are not individually appropriate.

When I reached menopause in the early 1990s, I refused to worry about my bones. After all, I had been paying attention to food and health for more than thirty years, and I felt that was enough. I got interested in vegetarianism in my teens, in macrobiotics in my twenties, started to teach natural foods cooking in my thirties, and branched out into offering classes on how food affects our health and well-being in general. In the process of teaching about everything that I wanted to learn, I founded The Natural

Gourmet Cookery School, and its sister institution, The Natural Gourmet Institute for Food and Health. As I like writing as much as teaching, I wrote two cookbooks: *The Book of Whole Meals,* which showed how to organize breakfasts, lunches, and dinners based on whole grains and beans, which first came out in 1979; and *The Natural Gourmet,* with some more adventuresome recipes and menus based on the Chinese Five Phase Theory, published in 1989. In between, I wrote what I call my "think-book," *Food and Healing,* published in 1986 and reissued in 1996 for a tenth anniversary edition. *Food and Healing* is my attempt to lay out a unified theory of how food affects our health, which then provides the basis for us to choose the healthiest foods in many different circumstances, and to avoid getting trapped in food ideologies that get us boxed in too rigidly.

As I paid attention to the lessons taught me by my life, my family, my children, my students, and many other people who shared and discussed their experiences with me, I slowly kept changing my teaching, adding and subtracting ideas, until I came full circle and saw the benefits of many different, natural foods, both of plant and of animal origin. I found people who do well on vegetarian or vegan diets, and others who need not just fish but even red meat in their diets to function optimally. I found many people, including myself and my children, who do better without milk products and sugar, and others who do well eating some cheese or yogurt. What did not vary was my view that people also need plenty of vegetables and whole grains, and that the best foods are invariably those that nature provides: whole, fresh, natural, *real* foods. I believe strongly that in a healthy diet there is no place for factory-formulated, artificially colored, flavored, sweetened, or otherwise fake foods. I found that any diet that focuses on just one of the macronutrients—protein, carbohydrates, or fats—either to enhance or to eliminate it, sooner or later turns out to be imbalanced or insufficient. The secret, as we all know, is in finding the food that balances our lives. More than anything, I believe that in order to be healthy, we need to pay attention to how we're doing every day, not just when we get sick. In the same way we keep our homes clean and our cars running with the proper amount of oil and gas, we need to keep our bodies clean inside as well as out, and give them the proper amount of appropriate foods and fluids so we can live and be useful and happy.

Publisher Elaine Koster of Dutton Signet knew about my work, and when she asked me to write a book on food and osteoporosis, I was flattered but hesitant. After all, I wasn't paying attention to the issue other than having figured out what my basic view of it was. But then I became intrigued, and the more I researched it the more fascinated I got. The subject turns out to be immensely complex. Our bones, after all, are not just the support system for our muscles and organs. Christiane Northrup, M.D., the author of *Women's Bodies, Women's Wisdom*, pointed out to me in a conversation that, metaphorically, our bones represent our core and our connection to the earth. As we lose that connection, our bones suffer. Women suffer more than men, Dr. Northrup said, because traditionally women have been the keepers of connection with the earth.

We all know that deep meaning of our skeleton. When we get a hunch, we say, "I feel it in my bones." When we want to express the deepest pain, we say, "It hurts all the way through to my bones." When the bones become brittle, therefore, it could mean that our entire life's framework lacks support. I believe that our current concern with bones, and the widely reported problem of osteoporosis, indicates that something is missing in the basic structure of our lives. Whatever is missing in each of us can only be found individually. Becoming conscious of it is the first step. The next step is to attend to strengthening the physical structure, and at the same time, to look ever deeper into ourselves and strengthen our spirit. Let us attend, then, not only to the physical aspect of our skeleton, but to its metaphorical aspects as well.

This book looks at both, with the mission of giving you a better understanding and some practical tools. Its main focus, however, is on how food affects bone health, which foods weaken it, and how smart food choices can strengthen it and prevent osteoporosis. In addition, these balanced and nutritious food choices will strengthen your entire body; as the song says, "the foot bone's connected to the ankle bone, the ankle bone's connected to the leg bone," and all the bones are connected to each other and to everything else. Eating well is the best preventive medicine.

I hope you will find some ideas here that apply to you, to help you remain strong until the day you decide to leave the earth. Once you know the facts, your own individual course of action will become clearer. The recipes included at the end of the book will get you started. Let's remember that, after the body dies, the bones could remain intact for millennia—if they can last that long we should be able to keep them from weakening and breaking while we are alive!

New York City
September 1997

1

Defining the Problem

To every action there is an equal and opposite reaction.
—Sir Isaac Newton

My Experience with Osteoporosis

Though I haven't experienced the effects of osteoporosis myself, I can share with you some personal observations about women and their risk for fractures, especially when older.

First, my mother. She died in 1991, at the age of eighty-six, and was most of her life quite healthy. Even at an advanced age, she never suffered from any illness except progressive deafness. I believe what harmed her the most was a car accident she suffered at the age of eighty-one, where she was thrown from the car she was driving and was given up for dead. She recuperated, but the blow to her head appeared to have started a senility process that took her downhill.

Even with the accident and several falls in the street, she never broke a single bone. She also didn't seem to shrink much as she aged, and wasn't stooped over. Thus I assume she didn't suffer from osteoporosis. The aspects of her life that I find meaningful in this respect are these:

- She had watched her diet for forty years, eating mostly whole grains and whole-grain bread, vegetables, salads, fruit, with small amounts of fish, chicken, and rarely some meat. On the whole, she avoided white flour and sugar. On birthdays and outings she would indulge in sweets, but not otherwise. Her main dietary "sin" as she called it, was coffee, which she often tried to give up but always returned to. (I, who am not a coffee drinker, couldn't understand why she had so much trouble with it; when I asked her why she didn't drink tea instead, she dismissed the idea with a hand wave. "Bah," she said, "too wimpy.")

- While she did eat the occasional potato, her major source of starches were whole-grain bread and brown rice, and sometimes beans. (If this makes you think that she was a woman ahead of her time, you are right. It also shows you where I came from: she was the one who taught me.)

- She never took any type of medication, either over the counter or prescribed. Her physician was a homeopath, whom she hardly ever visited. She felt that most of the diseases of older people are a result of the drugs and medicines they take.

- She walked a lot. Whenever she came to visit me in New York, already in her seventies, she would regularly walk forty or fifty blocks daily.

Another person who influenced my observations is my aunt (who was actually my mother's cousin and one year younger). She died in 1997, six months before turning ninety. She had also never broken a bone. What I saw in her was an interesting progression with weight. She was of normal weight all her life until menopause, when she put on about thirty pounds. By the time she turned eighty, she had lost the weight, and was beginning to look really thin. Her health was quite good, and she only complained about her fading eyesight.

Both my mother and my aunt lived in Argentina since the late 1940s, and I returned to visit yearly from 1988. One year when I returned and my aunt was about eighty-four, I noticed that she had become very thin and bowlegged, a condition she had never had before; her knees also hurt on the outside. She was living alone at the time, and eating little. Like my mother, she used no medications, and her diet was semivegetarian, but she ate many more nightshade vegetables and white bread. Eventually I arranged for her to live with a caretaker, who fed her abundantly and eventually helped her put on about twenty pounds. I also instructed that her intake of potatoes and tomatoes be curtailed. The following year, I found that her legs had gotten stronger and the pain in her knees had disappeared.

Reflecting on these observations, I realized that the women I know who have broken bones after menopause generally shared two or more of the following characteristics:

- Their diet was rich in meats, white flour, sugar, potatoes, and tomatoes.
- They didn't hesitate to take pharmaceutical medicines, either over the counter or prescribed.
- They didn't do much exercise.
- They were thin, either because they didn't eat enough or because they dieted to stay that way.

Neither my mother nor my aunt took hormone replacements, calcium supplements, or any other supplements or vitamins. They both had the same disdain for pills, and I have surely inherited it. They did eat some dairy foods, both having been born in Holland, but only by consuming cheese or yogurt occasionally. They didn't drink milk regularly, or eat ice cream except as a rare treat.

Because of my observations and experiences, I do not believe that the current approach to preventing or treating osteoporosis with drugs, pills, and milk products is the right way to go. After all, one of the most interesting epidemiological aspects of the condition is that it occurs more in cities and in "first world" countries where these practices are common, rather than in rural areas and "third world" countries where they are not. Specifically, it occurs more in the European and North American countries where people eat large amounts of milk products than in the African countries where people eat almost none.

A Personal Philosophy

In order to make good decisions and choices, we need a basic philosophy that directs us, that is cohesive enough so that our choices have the desired results. Otherwise we are at the mercy of other people telling us what to do based on *their* philosophy. For example, if we are told that calcium pills prevent osteoporosis, the underlying assumption is that

- pills are a valid way to help us keep our health,
- they are better and/or more convenient than food,
- the only effect they will have is the intended one.

If that is our own assumption as well, then taking calcium pills is harmonious with our belief system. On the other hand, if our belief system is that

- pills are a poor way to maintain health,
- the natural world gives us better choices,
- there are always adverse effects from pills,

then it makes no sense within that viewpoint to take the pills.

Perhaps I oversimplify. Certainly there are many who do not share my viewpoint. As physician Mark Liponis commented to me, "Your belief in nature's perfection may be appropriate with perfect genes and perfect conditions. I have seen so many instances of nature's imperfections that I have a somewhat different philosophy." Fair enough. No matter what our philosophy is, we'll all be right in some cases and wrong in others. I am reminded of a quote once from a doctor addressing a class of medical students: "Remember that half of what you learn in medical school is wrong. The difficulty is in finding out which half."

You need to know what your own underlying belief system is. I cannot discern that. What I will do here is share my own, so that you know why I make the choices that I make. Once you know where I stand, you can also make your own decisions better, either by agreeing or disagreeing with mine. Follow me, then, while we take a short detour into a philosophy of life.

The Movement of Life Energy

Energy moves between opposite poles; every action has its consequences. I believe that life works like a seesaw, or a pendulum swing. So, in fact, did Newton, who made this concept one of the pillars of his physical laws, and so do many systems of thought throughout history: action and reaction, up and down, night and day. These are all *sets of opposites*, like the two sides of the coin, and just as inseparable. Right and wrong, yin and yang are two of the better-known social constructs on this theme. For the past five thousand years *right and wrong* has been the basic mode of thought of the Western hemisphere, while *yin and yang* has been the foundation of Chinese thought.

The main difference between those two viewpoints is in their judgment. "Right and wrong" implies that if one part is good or right, the other automatically has to be bad or wrong—and often that is taken to mean that the "opposite" has to be eliminated. "Yin and yang" are simply nonjudgmental descriptions, no superiority of one over the other is implied, and no destruction of one or the other is required. When we deal with right and wrong, or good and bad, and eliminate one of the parts of the "set" (the one considered *wrong* or *bad*), it's like "cutting off your nose to spite your face." *Trying to eliminate one part of the set of opposites ("action") will negatively affect the other part of this set of opposites ("reaction").* This is a universal law and cannot be escaped. Example: Early this century it was decided that mosquitoes were a bad thing because they brought malaria. It was decided that mosquitoes should be eradicated, and DDT was used liberally in the service of that viewpoint. This was action. What was the reaction? Not only did the mosquitoes die, but the birds died as well, poisoned by the pesticide. In fact, the whole earth got poisoned, and it still is.

Life does not proceed in a straight line; it curves and sends us curveballs. No one has said that better, in my opinion, than Richard Grossinger in his fine book *Planet Medicine*:

> "Purposeful behavior itself is often counterproductive. In seeking immediate goals, men generate unending secondary consequences in the natural and cosmic systems of which they are part, a system which is more complex and subtle than their intentions."

For all these reasons, I don't like pills and drugs. They always have "unending secondary consequences," and those are usually difficult to anticipate. This makes me a rather antisocial member of our society, as our culture impresses upon us the desirability and the need to take pills and drugs for a variety of ills, particularly the ills of women. Money is not a small part of what makes this system run.

I know I am not alone in this viewpoint. Many people say, "I don't like taking things"—I hear that often—however, they generally follow it with "but I don't know what else to do," and a sigh. The medical model we live by relies greatly on man-made substances to maintain or enhance our health, either in pill form, or in the form of syrups, drops, and injections. Most people are so used to this model that they find it often hard to expand their belief system or change their habits of "taking something." They find it hard to believe that anything else can have a positive effect, and their instinct that "doesn't like taking things" is ignored in favor of the social medical mores.

Another aspect of this philosophy of life is trust in the life process, trust that the body has its reasons that reason does not understand. The body's job is staying alive day in and day out, knowing what to do with air, food, and water, sleeping and waking. We are born with this knowledge. It is part and parcel of each one of us. When things go wrong, I believe it is important to work *with* the body's knowledge, to listen carefully to what it tells us, and provide what's missing or remove what's in excess. This is what the natural healing model proposes to do. The medical model tends to work *against* the body—witness the list of "anti" medications: antibiotics, anti-inflammatories, ant(i)acids, and the like. The adverse effects are inevitably reactions of the body to being pulled in directions in which it doesn't want to go.

My view is that the natural healing model is more accurate and has better results for disorders of function, that is, to deal with the body that isn't doing things "right." Western medicine is best to deal with problems of structure, or mechanical issues; in fact, nothing comes close to its ability to save lives in emergencies like car crashes, burns, gunshot wounds. Drugs, on the other hand, are a different story. *All* man-made drugs or supplements have unbalancing or adverse effects: they are a double-edged sword. They have desired effects, and they also have adverse effects. Both kinds are equal. Both "count." We cannot have one without the other. When we rely on drugs for most of our health needs, the adverse effects must be taken into account at all times. For osteoporosis in particular, which seriously affects about 40 to 50 percent of postmenopausal women, numerous medications, supplements, and drugs are regularly recommended as prevention of fractures. Using drugs to prevent something that may *or may not* happen (50 to 60 percent of postmenopausal women *do not* get osteoporotic fractures) could cause adverse effects that may be worse than the problem presumably avoided. We need to assess carefully the risks of taking these drugs before jumping into the Pied Piper line set up by good marketing companies.

The axiom "the benefits outweigh the risks" is true of drugs mostly in life-threatening cases. If the choice is between suffocating from an asthma attack and losing a little bone mass from the steroids, the choice is fairly clear. But if the choice is between shrinking a little less and an increased risk of breast cancer associated with hormone replacement therapy, I can't see it.

I know there are many people who, in greater or lesser form, believe as I do. This book, then, is about keeping our bones strong without taking drugs or pills, so as to avoid the "unending secondary consequences" and deal simply with the problem as it is. Let's now take a look at the basic facts of the problem.

2

What Is Osteoporosis?

My bones consumed away through my daily complaining.
—Psalms 32:3

The bones that compose the skeleton keeping us upright are living, moving tissue. Like the shroud woven by Penelope, the wife of Odysseus, they are continuously being built up and broken down. Osteoporosis is a condition in which normally dense bone tissue has become less dense, showing holes and spaces. This happens when the buildup of bone is not keeping pace with the breakdown, and the bone's protein structure and mineral content are lost. If the condition continues to progress, bone mass becomes lower and lower, the bones become more porous, weaker, and lighter, and the risk of fracture increases.

Why Is Osteoporosis a Health Issue?

Some bone loss, between 0.5 and 1.5 percent a year, is a normal part of aging, and may pose no problem. Porous bones themselves are not dangerous, nor do they cause any symptoms. The main issue is the risk of fracture, especially in the elderly. Not all fractures are caused by osteoporosis—car or ski accidents and falls from heights can cause fractures, even in people with strong bones—but in many cases a fracture is the first sign of thinning bones.

It is estimated that more than 25 million people in the United States are affected by this condition. Some 40 percent of women and 13 percent of men may sustain a fracture after age 50. More than 1.3 million fractures annually are attributed to osteoporosis. Among them are some 500,000 vertebral or spine fractures, 250,000 hip fractures, and 240,000 wrist fractures. The numbers are different in different countries: reported incidences of hip fractures are highest in the United States and Northern Europe, intermediate in Mediterranean and Asian countries, and lowest in South Africa, particularly in the areas where people follow traditional ways of life. There are more fractures among city dwellers than among country folk. Over the past forty or fifty years, the incidence of hip fractures seems to have risen significantly in a number of countries. In addition, the incidence of hip fractures rises 30-fold between the ages of fifty and eighty.

Hip fractures are serious business. About half of those who sustain a hip fracture become temporarily or permanently disabled from ensuing complications such as blood clots or pneumonia; some 20 percent may require long-term nursing care, and about 20 percent may die within a year. Other bone fractures are also associated with at least temporary pain and disability. Vertebral or spinal fractures cause deformities of the spine, the hunched-over "dowager's hump" condition, and loss of height.

What Causes Osteoporosis?

Contrary to popular wisdom, lack of calcium is not the only cause of osteoporosis. According to researchers Giorgio Cotrozzi and Patrizia Relli of the Istituto di Clinica Medica at the Universita degli Studi of Florence, Italy, osteoporosis can be classified in the following general types according to their possible causes:

Primary Osteoporosis

Postmenopausal osteoporosis (type I). Lower estrogen levels in postmenopausal women cause a lessening of bone mass over time, starting at about 3 percent for the first year and then diminishing to 1.5 to 2 percent yearly. There are considerable individual variations: ten years after the menopause some women have lost only 5 to 10 percent of their bone mass, while others have lost as much as 40 percent.

Senile osteoporosis (type II). Advancing age, particularly from the seventh decade onward, brings a lower absorption of calcium from the intestine as well as a lower secretion of calcitonin, the hormone that prevents calcium from leaving the bones.

Secondary Osteoporosis

Endocrine osteoporosis. This occurs as a consequence of various disorders of the endocrine glands, such as the thyroid, the parathyroid, and the adrenal glands, all of which are involved in bone formation. Even diabetes, a disorder of the pancreas, another endocrine gland, can cause osteoporosis because it creates problems with the metabolism of vitamin D which helps absorb calcium from the intestines.

Sedentary osteoporosis. Caused by the lack of physical activity or by bed rest, which among other factors diminishes the intestinal absorption of calcium.

Malnutrition. Bones may suffer because of the lack of calories or nutrients in the diet, such as calcium, magnesium, various vitamins, fat, or protein.

Other Illnesses. Diseases of the liver, gastrointestinal tract, kidneys, as well as various cancers including bone cancer may have a secondary effect on bone formation and contribute to weakness or fractures.

Iatrogenic. A number of pharmacological drugs (corticosteroids, anticoagulants, antiepileptic drugs, certain diuretics, lithium, antitumor agents, thyroid hormones) are known to cause bone loss.

If you have been told that you have or are at risk for osteoporosis, do any of the above apply to you?

Who Gets Osteoporosis?

Both women and men may get this condition. In this country, it is found in about twenty million women and about five million men. Men suffer about one-half the hip fractures and one-sixth the spinal fractures of women. About 25 to 30 percent of postmenopausal women suffer major orthopedic problems because of osteoporosis.

The generally accepted risk factors for the condition in women include the following:

- Being small-boned, of European or Asian descent
- Postmenopause, natural or surgical
- Family history of hip fractures
- No natural children

For men, who have been studied much less in this regard, the risk factors include:

- Testosterone insufficiency
- Advanced age

For both sexes, the following risk factors apply:

- Delayed puberty
- Alcohol consumption
- Smoking
- Sedentary life, lack of exercise
- Thinness or being noticeably underweight
- Malnutrition
- Insufficient peak bone mass around age thirty
- Insufficient calcium
- Insufficient vitamin D
- Use of corticosteroids or other medical drugs
- Thyroid or kidney disorders
- Malignancies (multiple myeloma, bone cancer)
- Gastrointestinal diseases (inflammatory bowel disease, gastrectomy, gastric bypass, cirrhosis of the liver)

Based on my observations and understanding of food and lifestyle, in my view there are other significant dietary risk factors that have received insufficient attention:

- Eating a high proportion of animal protein together with flour products and sweets
- Eating a high proportion of nightshade vegetables (potatoes, tomatoes, eggplant, peppers)
- Not eating enough vegetables

- Not including enough good-quality fats in the diet
- Not including enough protein in the diet

Both too much and too little protein can cause trouble with the bones. Vegetarians have been shown to have higher bone density than omnivores, or people who eat everything (and presumably much more animal protein, but perhaps also less plant foods). In one study published in the *American Journal of Clinical Nutrition*, the mean bone density of the seventy- to seventy-nine-year-old vegetarians was greater than that of the fifty- to fifty-nine-year-old omnivores. Therefore, it is considered that vegetarians have a lesser risk of osteoporosis. Another way to interpret these studies is to note the rest of the dietary context: it could mean that the "omnivores" eat too many sweets and not enough greens and other plant foods. A 1997 Norwegian study found that there was an elevated risk of fracture in women with a high intake of protein *and a low calcium intake*.

We have heard that women who get pregnant may lose calcium from their own bones to provide it for the developing child. However, Nature does not abandon mothers. Women who have borne children appear to have a lower rate of bone loss *after* menopause than those who were never pregnant. This may be related to the increased level of calcitonin, the hormone that slows down bone resorption, which is increased in pregnant women and protects their bones from the fetal calcium drain.

It is generally assumed that low bone density indicates fracture risk. However, it looks as if dense bones may not necessarily be sufficient to prevent hip fractures if there are other risk factors. A 1995 study of sixty-five-year-old women, by Dr. Steven R. Cummings of the University of California at San Francisco, found a number of risk factors more significant than thin bones. They included:

- Taking tranquilizers and sleeping pills
- Smoking
- Having vision problems such as poor depth perception
- A past history of having an overactive thyroid gland
- Being tall
- Being unable to get out of a chair without holding onto the arms
- Having a high pulse rate

Women who had five or more of these risk factors—*regardless of bone density!*—had a 10 percent chance of breaking a hip in the next five years, while those with two or less risk factors only had a 1 percent chance of doing so. In addition, it was found that smoking is a particularly noxious risk factor: smokers were thinner, in poorer health, less likely to walk for exercise, and had faster heart rates than nonsmokers, all factors that would increase their chances of falling and breaking a hip.

That bone density is misleading is well known to those who pay attention. In 1996, the National Women's Health Network organized a panel discussion on estrogen replacement therapy. One finding was that low bone density is not a good predictor of bone fractures; better predictors are advanced age accompanied by poor muscle strength, the use of regular medications such as tranquilizers, barbiturates, sleeping pills, thyroid replacement therapy, and corticosteroids, as well as impaired vision. The benzodiazepine drugs, in fact, have been found to increase the risk of hip fracture by 70 percent, according to a Canadian study published in the *Journal of the American Medical Association* in 1989.

So we can see that low bone density is only one of the many risk factors for bone fracture. "We know that many people with osteoporosis never break their hips, and some with normal bone density do," says Mark Liponis, M.D., a physician at Canyon Ranch in the Berkshires. "That has a lot to do with activity level, reflexes, 'padding,' sensory impairment, balance, agility and the tendency to fall, as well as the use of sedatives or alcohol."

Defining the Problem

Osteoporosis is a condition when both protein and mineral are lost from bone, showing more holes and spaces. The risk of fracture is increased.

Causes: malnutrition, sedentary life, advanced age, hormonal insufficiency (estrogen, testosterone, thyroid, adrenal hormones), illness (including cancer), drugs (steroids, diuretics).

Major risk factors (for men or women): advanced age, alcohol consumption, smoking, lack of exercise, thinness or being underweight, use of pharmacological drugs, diet high in protein, flour, and sweets, diet lacking vegetables, fats, protein, high consumption of nightshade vegetables (potatoes, tomatoes, peppers, eggplant).

It is clear that the problem of osteoporosis is highly complex. Swallowing a few calcium tablets as prevention may not be enough and may in fact be counterproductive: the Nurses Health Study found that dietary calcium exceeding 450 mg per day actually doubled the risk of hip fracture. We need a radical change in outlook.

3
Looking at Bones

*Thou knowest not what is the way of the spirit, nor how
the bones do grow in the womb of her that is with child.*
—Ecclesiastes 11:5

Some of our major problems in life result when we get involved in doing
things without having a good grasp of what is going on. This is particularly
true of medical issues. But while we've been trained to just do what the
doctor says, that attitude is changing today. Many of us are no longer willing to take a pat on the head and be told, "Trust me, dear." As educated
people, we want things explained and we want to be able to make judg-
ments and appropriate choices. Even if we do end up doing as we're told,
we want to do it out of choice, not coercion.

To understand what the various osteoporosis prevention therapies pur-
port to do, we need to understand the details of what goes on in our bones.
Let's take a look at the basic facts.

How Bones Develop

How bones develop from a few cells is, like life in general, quite miracu-
lous. In the embryonic stage, they start off as cartilage, something similar
to a very firm gel, taking the same shape as the future bones. The cartilagi-
nous skeleton is completely formed at the end of the first trimester of preg-
nancy. Specialized cells in the center of the long bones, in the *diaphysis* or
"shaft," start actual bone formation growing toward the ends, or the *epiphyses*, while cells there also begin to ossify, or turn into bone. By the time

the baby is born, the bones have hardened most of the way, except for a disk of cartilage between the shaft and the epiphyses. This disk is called the *epiphyseal disk* or *growth disk*, and it allows the bones to keep growing until between the ages of 14 and 20, the different bones slowly ossify and fuse the gap to halt growth.

Also during embryonic life, the center of the long bones becomes hollowed out to make room for the cylindrical *marrow cavity*. In the adult skeleton, the walls around the marrow cavity are dense, hard, and compact, and called, appropriately, *compact bone*. The epiphyses, as well as the vertebrae, pelvis, and ribs are not so dense, and contain strands of bone that crisscross haphazardly, called *trabecular bone*; in between these strands there is red bone marrow, which forms red and white blood cells. At birth the marrow in the long bones is red as well, but eventually this is replaced with yellow marrow, which consists of minerals, connective tissue, and fat cells.

What Bones Are Made Of

Bones are composed of a latticed protein grounding or *collagen matrix*, which comprises about 35 percent of the bone and which gives it its flexibility. This matrix then traps the mineral salt *calcium phosphate*, which occupies about 65 percent of the bone mass and which gives the bone its strength. However, even though strong and hard, bones are not the equivalent of stones or rocks. Instead, like the rest of the tissues in the body, they are constantly moving and changing. They are continuously being built up, in a process called *deposition* or *formation*, and just as continuously being broken down, a process called *resorption*. About 5 to 10 percent of bone is replaced yearly in this fashion. From birth until sometime in our twenties, bone is built up faster than it is broken down. Between ages twenty-five and thirty, it is considered that we have reached "peak bone mass," and from then on bone resorption is slightly higher than deposition. At first, we may lose around 0.5 to 1 percent of bone per year. After menopause, bone loss may accelerate to between 1.5 and 5 percent per year, depending on a woman's nutrition, exercise, pharmacological drug intake, and overall health.

Being rich in calcium and hardness is not enough to make bones resistant to fracture. Bones can be dense yet brittle, lacking flexibility, which will cause them to break easily. The collagen matrix is crucial for maintaining flexibility, and may be more essential to preventing fractures than calcium content. In laboratory studies, if a bone is put in an acid bath and all the calcium is removed, it can then be bent and twisted like a tendon; it does not break. On the other hand, a dense, highly mineralized bone that has the collagen matrix diminished can break with slight pressure, or shatter under a sharp blow. For this reason, the tests that measure bone density will not accurately predict the risk for fracture. There are cases of women with demonstrated low bone mineralization, who in spite of repeated falls never break a bone: that is because their bones are *flexible*.

Bones are a reservoir of numerous other minerals that our bodies need for their day-to-day function, besides calcium. For that reason, the remodeling process is essential to our general health. Our bones, in fact, act a little like a "bank." Nutrients come and go as a continuous "cash flow" of "income" and "expenses." Calcium is the major element in this flow, together with phosphorus, sodium, magnesium, and protein.

The Role of Calcium

Calcium is the most abundant mineral in the body, and is absolutely essential for many physiological functions. Bones contain about 99 percent of all the calcium in the body; the rest is used throughout the body in functions such as blood clotting, nerve transmission, muscle contraction and growth, heart function, general metabolism, and various hormone functions. In the bones, the calcium is found in the form of *calcium phosphate salts*, not as pure calcium. About 85 percent of the body's phosphorus is stored in the bones. The ratio of calcium (Ca) to phosphorus (P) in these salts is 2.5 to 1. In addition to the calcium and phosphorus, our bones also store between 40 and 60 percent of our body's total sodium and magnesium.

Let's remember that if a little is good and a deficiency is bad, a lot is not necessarily better; in fact, a lot can be bad too. Lack of enough calcium prevents bone deposition and contributes to thinner bones. Too much calcium can encourage kidney stones and gallstones. Insufficient phosphorus prevents the body from creating the necessary calcium salts and weakens the bones; excess phosphorus in the form of phosphoric acid (found mainly in soft drinks, preservatives, and meats) can stimulate the release of calcium from the bones and thereby weakens them as well.

How Calcium Travels

The source of both calcium and phosphorus are the foods we eat. First, these foods are broken down in the stomach and duodenum, the upper part of the small intestine; then, as the food travels through the remaining twenty or so feet of it, the minerals are absorbed through the walls of the small intestine straight into the bloodstream. Once in the blood, the calcium can go straight to the bones and be deposited there for storage. Bone resorption takes place as needed, liberating calcium for necessary functions in the blood, muscles, nerves, heart muscle, and elsewhere. Excess calcium that does not go back into the bones gets excreted by the kidneys. Some calcium also remains unabsorbed in the undigested parts of the food and gets excreted.

Since we're comparing the bones to a bank, we need all kinds of helpers (tellers, accountants) to get the money (calcium) from here to there, and can encounter all manner of systems that check excessive growth (fees, taxes). What is the main helper element that keeps this input/output system moving? It's activity. Movement, walking, and the influence of gravity all help the deposition of calcium in the bones. It is well known that sedentary living, being bedridden, and weightlessness (such as that experienced by the astronauts in space), all contribute to the loss of bone mass. Lack of use prevents the deposition of calcium salts, so that the process of mineral resorption slowly uses up the available bone mass. In other words, "Use it or lose it!"

Main Elements of Bone Formation

In addition to calcium, there are other nutrients and elements that, as helpers, have a crucial influence on how bone is formed and resorbed. Here are the main elements that affect bone formation:

- Protein and vitamin C: Stimulate collagen matrix formation
- Vitamin D: Increases Ca absorption from small intestine into blood
- Magnesium: Increases Ca absorption from blood into bone
- Strain, stress, exercise, and movement: Increase bone deposition
- Sexual hormones (estrogens and progesterone, the female hormones; androgens, the male hormones): Increase bone deposition
- Thyroid and Parathyroid hormones: Calcitonin hormone secreted by the thyroid decreases bone resorption by slowing down or halting the

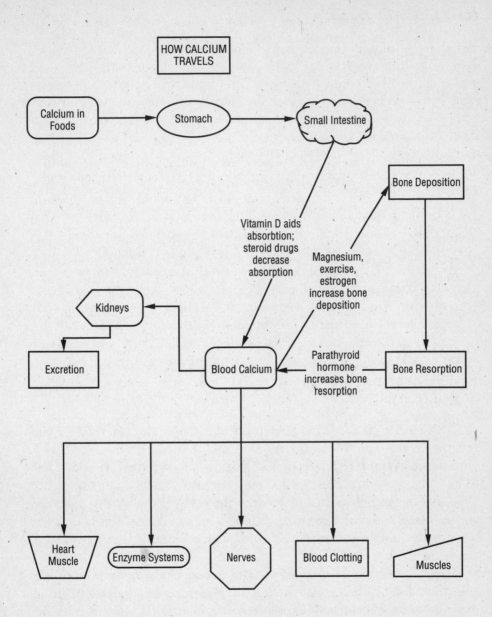

HOW CALCIUM TRAVELS

Calcium in Foods → Stomach → Small Intestine

Vitamin D aids absorbtion; steroid drugs decrease absorption

Magnesium, exercise, estrogen increase bone deposition

Bone Deposition

Kidneys → Excretion

Parathyroid hormone increases bone resorption

Blood Calcium ← Bone Resorption

Heart Muscle — Enzyme Systems — Nerves — Blood Clotting — Muscles movement of calcium out of the bones, decreasing blood Ca. Parathyroid hormone increases bone resorption by pulling Ca out of bones, increasing blood Ca.

Let's look at each of these factors.

Protein and Vitamin C

The formation of collagen is dependent on sufficient protein in the diet, as well as vitamin C, which stimulates the enzymes that form the collagen and connective tissue. A deficiency of either one could weaken the bone matrix, interfering with its ability to hold on to the calcium salts. Protein is found most abundantly in meats, fowl, fish, eggs, beans, nuts and seeds, as well as in lesser amounts in whole grains. Vitamin C is found in all fruits and vegetables; it does break down quickly in the presence of heat or oxygen, so the fresher the food the better. People who eat carelessly, focusing on carbohydrates and ignoring vegetables and protein, may be risking weak bones from collagen matrix insufficiency. Calcium supplements in these cases may be counterproductive: an excess of calcium and a lack of collagen matrix could make the bone hard but brittle, and so easily breakable.

Vitamin D

This nutrient is needed to help in absorbing calcium from the small intestine, as well as in the assimilation of phosphorus. This fat-soluble vitamin is actually more like a hormone, as it is synthesized by the body itself. The action of sunlight on the skin oils prompts its formation, and then it is absorbed through the skin back into the body. It can also be absorbed from food through the intestines in the company of essential fatty acids. The body stores significant reserves of this vitamin in the liver, spleen, bones, and brain.

Vitamin D_3, the natural form, also called cholecalciferol, is found mostly in fish oils. (It can also be made synthetically by ultraviolet light irradiation of a derivative of cholesterol.) Vitamin D_2 is a synthetic form, known as ergocalciferol. The vitamin D added to milk, a practice begun in the 1930s to prevent rickets, can be either one of those two synthetic forms.

The Recommended Daily Allowance is 400 IU (International Units). Doses of vitamin D_2 in excess of 1200 IU can be seriously toxic, causing calcification of soft tissues and of the walls of the blood vessels, heart tissues, lungs, and kidney tubules, a condition known as *hypercalcemia* or *milk-alkali syndrome*. In one unusual case in New England in the early 1990s, reported in the *New England Journal of Medicine*, some infants developed this condition from excess vitamin D fortification of milk through error at the dairy: instead of the standard 400 IU per quart, the concentration in some samples went as high as 232,565 IU per quart. Hypercalcemia is a serious condition, as it can result in irreversible brain damage, calcium deposits in the soft tissues and organs, and arteriosclerosis, sometimes within a day or two of exposure.

The best source for natural vitamin D, which will prevent excesses, is daylight, or sunlight whenever possible. Some thirty minutes a day, two or three times a week, with the face, hands, and maybe arms out in the light is usually sufficient for most people. (For short exposures of this type, sun block is not advisable, as it keeps the beneficial light away from the skin and thereby interferes with vitamin D production.) Other good sources are fatty fish such as mackerel and salmon (make sure to eat the skin!), and even cod liver oil. There are vitamin D precursors in plant foods and leafy greens, known as *ergosterols*; parsley is a particularly rich source. While I have never seen this mentioned anywhere else, I found in my research for the recipes in this book that it is also abundant in shiitake mushrooms! (About 1 1/2 ounces, cooked, contain 69 percent of the RDA for a fifty-five-year-old woman.) Vitamin D can be destroyed in the intestines by mineral oil; therefore, when used as a laxative, this substance can interfere with calcium metabolism.

Magnesium

This nutrient is needed to stimulate the absorption of calcium into the bones. If there is a lack of magnesium, supplemental calcium may not go into strengthening the bones, but will remain in the bloodstream instead, perhaps contributing to kidney stones or gallstones. Nan Kathryn Fuchs, Ph.D., a nutritionist at The Health Center in Santa Monica, California, and columnist for the *Women's Health Letter*, points out that while magnesium helps the body absorb and utilize calcium, excessive calcium prevents the absorption of magnesium, and calcium without magnesium may create either calcium malabsorption or magnesium deficiency. Magnesium deficiency symptoms include hair loss, muscle contractions or cramps, nervous irritability, tremors, disorientation, and confusion.

Increasing magnesium intake *while lowering calcium intake to 500 milligrams per day* has been shown to increase bone density! Magnesium is found in whole grains, beans, fruits, and fresh vegetables; it is refined out of sugar, white flour, and white rice. Both sugar and alcohol cause magnesium to be excreted in the urine.

Perhaps you will be pleased to know that one of the foods highest in magnesium is chocolate, or cocoa powder. Is this an invitation to eat more chocolate? I wish. Unfortunately, the stimulants in chocolate, caffeine and theobromine, should give us pause. No, it just means that a craving for chocolate may indicate an underlying magnesium deficiency, which is best corrected with plenty of green vegetables, whole grains, and beans.

Strain, Stress, Exercise, and Movement

Movement against gravity helps deposit calcium salts in our bones. Walking is the most natural, most economical, and easiest way to insure continued bone health. Sedentary living, lots of sitting in chairs, cars, planes, and standing in elevators all contribute to bone weakness if not counteracted with enough appropriate activity and movement. We'll discuss this subject more fully in chapter 4.

Sexual Hormones

Estrogen and testosterone both promote the deposition of bone. For women undergoing menopause, the diminished production of estrogen promotes bone loss through lack of rebuilding. In other words, bone resorption continues, in order to satisfy the needs of the blood, muscles, heart, and nervous system for calcium and other minerals; but as deposition is less, bone density is lowered. A lack of androgens in men has also been shown to cause bone loss via the same process. The subject of estrogen replacement therapy will be discussed more fully in chapter 4 as well.

Thyroid and Parathyroid Hormones

Two hormones regulate the movement of calcium into and out of bone. The first is *calcitonin*, secreted by the thyroid gland below the Adam's apple in response to high amounts of calcium in the blood; this hormone lowers blood calcium by preventing bone resorption. The other hormone is *parathyroid hormone*, secreted by the four parathyroid glands that can be found on the four corners of the thyroid. The release of this hormone, triggered by below-normal levels of calcium in the blood, encourages bone resorption so as to raise those levels once again.

Other Necessary Nutrients

In addition to the minerals and vitamins already mentioned, nutritionist Ann Louise Gittleman, M.S., author of *Supernutrition for Menopause*, points out that we need the following nutrients to aid in bone building:

- Boron: for help in the synthesis of estrogen and vitamin D. It is found most abundantly in dried fruits and nuts.
- Manganese: essential for the utilization of vitamins B and C, for the synthesis of cartilage, and for bone growth and maintenance. Found mostly in nuts, seeds, whole grains, seaweed, and dark leafy greens.
- Vitamin K: necessary for blood clotting and the production of osteocalcin, which helps calcium crystallize in the bones and speeds the healing of fractures by stimulating bone growth. This vitamin is synthesized in the intestines by friendly bacteria, which can be destroyed by antibiotic use. Food sources include dark leafy greens, egg yolks, and fish-liver oils.
- Zinc: needed for normal bone formation by enhancing the action of vitamin D. Found mostly in meat, eggs, seafood, oysters, pumpkin seeds, and dried beans.
- Copper: essential for the formation of collagen. Food sources are organ meats, seafood, nuts, and seeds.
- Silicon: promotes the formation of bones and teeth, as well as collagen. Found in whole grains such as whole wheat, oats, and brown rice.
- Vitamin B_6 (pyridoxine): helps strengthen collagen. Best sources are bananas, carrots, onions, sunflower seeds, and walnuts, as well as whole grains.
- Folic acid: helps convert the amino acid homocysteine, which interferes with collagen synthesis, to the nontoxic form, cysteine. Best sources are leafy green vegetables, tuna, salmon, brown rice, beef, and beans.

This long list of nutrients that affect bone formation may be confusing, but let's be clear about one very important fact: the process of bone remodeling, the deposition of calcium salts, and the release of them back into the bloodstream to satisfy important metabolic needs is a careful set of checks and balances that keeps the system in equilibrium. Directly interfering with this balance, even when it looks like the body is doing its job incorrectly, should only be undertaken with extreme caution, if at all. I believe a better approach is to strengthen and nourish the body so it does its own healing. Nature knows what it's doing, and we often don't. In our ignorance, we try to "fix" things by direct action, where a more roundabout system could get better results. As bones are living tissue, it becomes clear that preventing fractures is a multifaceted endeavor. Alan R. Gaby, M.D., president of the American Holistic Medical Association and medical editor of *The Townsend Letter for Doctors*, points out in his book *Preventing and Reversing Osteoporosis* that to prevent fractures we need to pay attention "to at least three factors: 1) preventing loss of calcium and other minerals from bone; 2) maintaining the soft tissue components of bone, such as proteins, which give bones their unique structure; and 3) making sure that bones are capable of efficiently repairing damaged areas." That ability, of course, comes with a healthy body and strong immune system.

Looking at Bones

Bone composition: 35 percent is a latticed *collagen matrix*; 65 percent are *calcium phosphate salts*. Bones store 99 percent of the body's calcium, 85 percent of the phosphorus, and between 40 and 60 percent of the total body sodium and magnesium.
Bone remodeling: Bones are continuously being built up in a process called *deposition* or *formation*, and broken down in a process called *resorption*.
Major nutrients and other factors that help bone remodeling: Protein, vitamin C, vitamin D, magnesium, calcium, exercise and weight bearing, various hormones (estrogens, androgens, parathyroid hormone, calcitonin)
Also needed: Boron, manganese, vitamin K, zinc, copper, silicon, vitamin B_6, pyridoxine, folic acid

---

Now that we have a basic idea of what bones are, let's take a look at what can damage or weaken them from the inside.

4

What Weakens Our Bones

*Overindulgence in sweets will cause pain in the bones
and hair loss.*
— The Yellow Emperor's Classic of Internal Medicine

Here, of course, is the crux of the matter. How can we know what we should be doing about bone thinning, if we don't know what caused it? Wouldn't it be a waste of time and money to take calcium pills when what our body needs is magnesium? There are many variables in our contemporary lifestyle that contribute to osteoporosis. Let's take a look at them.

The Process of Bone Remodeling

The process of bone removal (resorption) and formation (deposition) is called *remodeling*. The ability of the bone to absorb and hold on to calcium salts is called *mineralization*. When both these processes slow down, bone mass decreases, and the condition is called *osteoporosis*, meaning a general loss of bone mass. When remodeling is abnormal and bone mass decreases, but the bone remaining has normal mineralization, the condition is called *osteopenia*. When mineralization is abnormal and bone mass decreases, the condition is called *osteomalacia*. If the mineralization is defective in growing bones, causing softness and bending, the condition is called *rickets*.

When they contain insufficient calcium salts, the bones become porous and soft; with insufficient protein or collagen, they become brittle. In osteoporosis there is a decrease in both, due to faulty remodeling (more is taken out than put in), so the bones become both porous *and* brittle. This

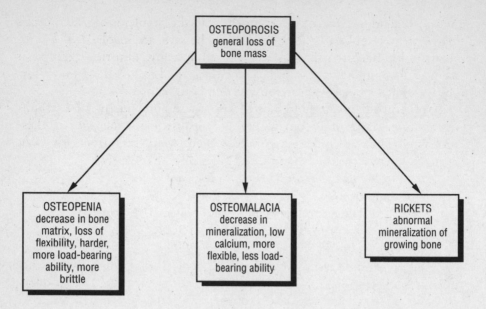

lack of building matter can be caused by a low supply of the necessary nutrients. However, a lack of nutrients is not the only cause: the highest incidence of osteoporosis is found in the United States and Scandinavia, countries that consume an abundance of milk products, which are high in both protein and calcium. In fact, a number of studies have failed to find a real connection between calcium intake and the risk of hip fracture. Something else must be at work here. It could be that the nutrients aren't absorbed. Or they could be drained or counteracted by other elements. Let's look at these possibilities.

Perhaps It's the Menopause

We hear this over and over again: once women grow older and their ovaries are producing less estrogen, bone loss inevitably follows and it's time for medication. I consider this a foolish notion. Turning the normal stages of a woman's life into medical conditions is a very popular pastime with the medical and drug establishments. To make the point better than I can, let me quote Professor John A. Kanis, from the World Health Organization Collaborating Centre for Metabolic Bone Diseases at the University of Sheffield Medical School in Great Britain. He writes in the journal

Bone: "The importance of the menopause to the problems of osteoporosis has been overemphasized." Other factors, he says, are involved in the increase in hip fracture risk that has occurred in many countries. The causes from this are unknown, but are clearly not related to just the menopause, "because these phenomena are observed in both men and women."

In other words, even though osteoporosis and bone fractures occur during the later stages of a woman's life, menopause is not the *cause* of these problems. They are only temporally related. More important for bone health is how we treat our bodies, and especially what we eat.

A Lack or a Drain?

What we eat both builds and fuels our bodies. Even though we have the notion that bones seem to just "sit there" and do nothing, the foods we consume affect them both directly and indirectly. Directly, because if we don't consume enough vitamin D, calcium, and protein, they will be unable to rebuild themselves. Indirectly, because as so many of the nutrients interrelate, the deficiency of one (vitamin D, for example) can cause a deficiency in another (calcium) even if there is enough quantity of the second in the diet. In addition, there are aspects of our diet that impact our bones because they cause an active calcium loss, or drain; over time, this drain can cause as much trouble as any nutrient deficiency.

Let's look at a concept that will help us understand the role of calcium and other minerals much more clearly: the acid-alkaline balance.

The Acid-Alkaline Balance

Perhaps you have heard of this concept. I have spent some time explaining it in my earlier books. I'll describe it again here, for it applies especially to the topic we are discussing.

Acids are substances containing hydrogen atoms that are missing electrons, so their tendency is to go steal electrons elsewhere: that thieving tendency makes them corrosive. In the body, acids generally result from metabolic processes such as moving or breathing; these acids are either excreted, or they're buffered (neutralized) by minerals or mineral salts, which in turn are considered alkaline (or *basic*). For the proper function of our metabolism, our blood plasma has to be slightly alkaline, at a pH of about 7.45 (a pH of 7 is neutral, below 7 is acid, above it is alkaline). This is a highly delicate balance, and going off even a little on either side can be fatal: for example, lockjaw, or tetany, precipitates an alkaline blood plasma pH of 7.9 and causes death; while diabetic coma accompanied by an acid pH of 6.9 also causes death. With a correct pH, the body is in *homeostasis*, or inner balance.

To keep the acid-alkaline (or acid-base) balance just right, the body has a number of mechanisms that increase or decrease both sides of the equation:

- Breathing: The cells breathe out carbonic acid, which becomes carbon dioxide and is expelled through the lungs, lowering the body's acid load.
- Moving: The movement of muscles creates lactic acid as it breaks down glycogen (stored carbohydrate) to produce energy, increasing the acid load.
- The kidneys regulate the acid-alkaline balance in the blood by excreting a more acid or more alkaline urine according to need.
- The foods we eat contribute to either an acid or an alkaline environment *once they're metabolized*. This depends on the residue they leave behind: they leave either acids (carbonic, phosphoric, or sulfuric) and therefore are *acid-forming*, or they leave buffering minerals (mostly calcium, iron, magnesium, potassium, sodium) and thereby are *alkalizing*.

Here is a simple concept to help you remember this model: the more minerals there are in a food, the more they alkalize the body. Protein and carbohydrate foods are acid-forming because they leave behind an acid residue; acid-forming foods include sugar, flour, beans, grains, fish, fowl, meat, and eggs. Most produce are alkalizing because they leave behind an alkaline residue in the form of minerals. Alkalizing foods include fruits, vegetables, sea vegetables, soy sauce, miso, and salt.

Acid-Forming and Alkalizing Foods

Acid-Forming Foods	Buffers	Alkalizing Foods
Alcohol	Yogurt	Juices
Sugar	Milk	Fruits
Oils	Cheese	Green vegetables
Nuts	Tofu	Green beans
Flour		Potatoes
Whole grains		Root vegetables
Beans		Sea vegetables
Fish		(seaweeds)
Fowl		Soy sauce
Meat		Miso
Eggs		Salt

The trick, of course, is to eat from both groups, and pick the healthier foods from each column. Eating too high a proportion of acid-forming foods will draw minerals out of the bones; while eating a high proportion of alkalizing foods often tends to create cravings for sweets, as many vegetarians will attest to.

The buffer foods are milk products and tofu (if made with calcium carbonate); they will balance either side, because they contain both calcium (alkalizing) and protein (acid-forming). Thus, if a diet is high in sugar, flour, and/or meats yet low in vegetables, dairy will help alkalize the body because of its calcium content. Conversely, if a diet is high in alkalizing fruits, vegetables, and potatoes yet low in protein or grains, dairy products will provide supplementary acid-forming protein.

For people who prefer not to use milk products, then, the solution is to consume instead plenty of dark green leafy vegetables (kale, collards, mustard greens, watercress, arugula), roots (carrots, turnips, parsnips, radishes), broccoli, squashes, and especially chopped parsley. Parsley contains both calcium and vitamin C, as well as ergosterol, a precursor to vitamin D, which helps absorb and utilize the calcium. I do not recommend spinach, even though it is rich in calcium, as it is also high in oxalic acid, which interferes with the absorption of calcium and thereby negates its value.

A slight tilt toward acidity in the bloodstream, called acidosis (or, if you will, a reduction of alkalinity), can remove calcium from the bones so as to neutralize it. Studies done on mice at the University of Rochester School of Medicine and Dentistry have shown that calcium does indeed leave the bones when they are in an acid environment. In other words, *metabolic acidosis stimulates bone resorption and inhibits bone formation.*

Dr. T. Colin Campbell of Cornell University, in collaboration with the Institute of Nutrition and Food Hygiene of the Chinese Academy of Preventive Medicine in Beijing, conducted a famous study of the dietary patterns and nutritional status in Chinese people in the early nineties. That study showed clearly that the composition of urinary acids and calcium in middle-aged and elderly women is influenced considerably by their dietary intakes. The consumption of acid-forming foods such as animal protein increased calcium excretion in the urine, which indicates bone mineral loss. Plant protein intake was not related to urinary calcium excretion. This finding may be one of the reasons why vegetarians have less osteoporosis than meat eaters. However, I am convinced that acidosis can also occur from too much flour or sugar. Metabolic acidosis from excess acid-forming foods in general would then have a *calcium-wasting* effect, or drain. The theory that protein foods such as red meat cause bone loss was debunked by the studies of Herta Spencer of the Veterans Administration Hospital in Hines, IL, in the 1980s. Dr. Spencer found that studies correlating calcium loss with high-protein diets used fractionated, isolated amino acids from milk or eggs; complex dietary proteins such as red meat did not cause calcium losses.

Must I Be a Vegetarian?

In the last quarter century we have focused on the excess of animal proteins in the diet, and found them damaging. Many studies of protein foods determined that their acid residue is bad for the bones. However, the observations of Weston Price, D.D.S., author of *Nutrition and Physical Degeneration*, shows that excellent bone health is found in traditional populations with diets high in fish and meats, as long as they also contain plenty of animal fats and vegetables. Dr. Price traveled all over the world in the early 1930s, and studied the health, dental health, and diet of traditional societies, all of which consume some animal protein. As other anthropologists before and after, he found no people subsisting on only plant foods, although these do make up a considerable percentage of native diets. He also found that traditional people often go through great trouble to get nutrient-rich fish, eggs, and other animal foods for pregnant women and those getting ready for parenthood.

The healthiest people that he found in terms of bones and teeth were six tribes in sub-Saharan Africa that subsisted mostly on the meat, milk, and blood of cows. These six cattle-herding tribes were completely free of cavities (0 percent decay), and had strong straight teeth and bones. The agricultural tribes, such as the Kikuyu and Wakamba, who consumed sweet potatoes, corn, beans, millet, and sorghum, plus small animals and insects, had decay in 5 to 6 percent of all teeth (in the United States as many as 75 percent of all teeth have tooth decay). However, Sally Fallon, editor of the *Health Journal* of the Price-Pottenger Nutrition Foundation, pointed out that the healthiest tribe Dr. Price found, the Sudanese Dinkas, lived on a diet consisting mainly of fish and cereal grains.

Although much attention has been paid to protein, refined carbohydrates have received relatively little notice, mostly because of the unfortunate viewpoint that "all carbohydrates are equal." Which they are not, as anyone who's tasted the difference between whole-grain and white bread can tell you. Christiane Northrup, M.D., pointed out to me that osteoporosis only appears in countries where the diet includes the habitual use of refined foods. Dr. Price, in fact, found countless cases of dental and skeletal defects (including caries, jaw malformations, and clubfeet) among traditional peoples who had switched to the "civilized" diet of white bread, sugar, jam, sweetened condensed milk, canned vegetables, and alcohol. The natives who remained on their traditional diet regardless of the amount of protein consumed were, on the other hand, found to be without these defects and in good health.

Calcium/Mineral Wasters (Drainers)

We know that a lack of "income" will lower our "bone assets"; but too many "expenses," using up what comes in and more, will do the same. Therefore, let's pay attention to the many different unhealthy ways in which we actually can remove more nutrients from our bones than we would under healthier conditions.

Refined Carbohydrates

As we've seen, acid-forming foods promote a tendency toward acidosis in the bloodstream; to counteract this acidosis, calcium and other minerals will be immediately withdrawn from the bones. Thus, bone resorption would increase to rebalance the blood, and calcium and other minerals would be excreted in the urine. An increase in alkalizing foods can balance this equation, by replacing the minerals that have been "borrowed" from the bones. However, if the diet is low in vegetables and other mineral-rich foods, and if this persists for year after year, the amount of calcium and other minerals needed for bone deposition ("income") would be too low, and slowly the "expenses" of bone resorption would exceed the "income."

Let's make no mistake: As their metabolic by-products include carbonic acid, carbohydrate foods are seriously acid-forming. Whole grains at least have some fiber, trace minerals, and vitamin E in them. Refined carbohydrates lack those natural nutrients, and thereby their ability to create an acidifying effect is enhanced, as they'll do little else. The regular consumption of white flour, white rice, and refined sugar will, therefore, contribute mightily to bone weakness; these are, without a doubt in my mind, probably your worst calcium-drainers. Perhaps that explains the high rates of osteoporosis in Western countries which, in addition to dairy and meats, also consume a high proportion of white bread, sweet snacks, and pastries.

Refined white sugar is particularly noxious, and by some perverse twist we have come to believe that sugar-sweetened desserts are essential to "having fun." We feed our children this devitalized food because they are socialized to expect it, and we to provide it. As adults, most people like to end their meals with a sugar-sweetened dessert, anything from ice cream to cake or cookies. The absence of such a dessert at an elegant dinner party would almost be a social faux pas.

What is so bad about this ubiquitous substance? According to nutritionist Robert Crayhon, author of *Nutrition Made Simple*, sugar can

- raise the insulin level and contribute to diabetes
- raise blood pressure, cholesterol, and triglycerides and so contribute to cardiovascular disease
- contribute to gallstones and obesity
- contribute to mood swings and depression
- increase stomach acidity
- cause migraines
- weaken the immune system
- deplete the B vitamins, calcium, and copper
- interfere with the absorption of calcium and magnesium—and so contribute to osteoporosis

But despite what we know about the substance British physician John Yudkin calls "sweet and dangerous" and "pure, white, and deadly," many people still feel that they might be "deprived" when they consider quitting the consumption of sugar-sweetened foods. I maintain that, for our long-term health, that's the kind of "deprivation" that would be a good thing, just like a deprivation of tobacco would be good too.

Caffeine

The consumption of caffeine is extremely common in our society. Most people rely on at least one cup of coffee in the morning to wake up. But caffeine is found in hundreds of other common foods and drinks, such as chocolate chip cookies, soft drinks, and even diet soft drinks, many of which one may not think of as containing caffeine.

As we'll see, caffeine can have a strong effect on our bones. It is found primarily in these four natural substances:

> coffee (regular, decaf)
> tea (black, green)
> chocolate
> mate *(MAH-tay)* (South American herbal tea)

Foods that contain caffeine either have one of the above as an ingredient or have had pure caffeine added, as is done with soft drinks and medications.

Where Caffeine Is Found (partial list)

regular coffee	dark chocolate	cola drinks
decaf coffee	milk chocolate	diet cola drinks
instant coffee	chocolate syrup	some other soft drinks
black tea	chocolate candy bar	some over-the-counter
instant tea	chocolate chip cookies	drugs and head-
iced tea	chocolate ice cream	ache remedies

How does this all relate to osteoporosis? It turns out that there are a number of studies that have shown that caffeine intake is related to both fractures and calcium depletion. A six-year-long study in the early eighties, completed at the Department of Medicine of Brigham and Women's Hospital in Boston, followed 84,484 women aged thirty-four to fifty-nine, and found that those with a higher caffeine intake (five or more cups of coffee daily) had an almost three times higher risk of hip fractures.

Caffeine consumption increases the excretion of calcium as well as magnesium through the urine, which indicates bone loss. Young women seem to be able to compensate for this loss and make it up faster through increased and more efficient calcium absorption from the intestines. Older women, on the other hand, with age- and hormone-related calcium imbalances, do not seem to be able to compensate as efficiently, and are at higher risk for thinning bones, especially if their calcium intake is low.

How high is a high-caffeine intake? According to a study done at the Department of Family and Preventive Medicine at University of California at San Diego, a lifetime equivalent of two cups of coffee per day is associated with decreased bone density at both the hip and the spine in older women if they don't also drink milk. (Moderate daily milk consumption, about one glass of milk per day, seems to counterbalance somewhat the calcium-wasting effect of caffeine.) The studies that I found all dealt with caffeinated coffee; I didn't find any on decaffeinated coffee, so I have no data on its effect on the bones. However, my suspicion is that decaf is not much better, as coffee is brewed from beans, which are acid-forming; besides, there still are traces of caffeine in the decaf. A study run by *Self* magazine in March 1996 found anywhere between 2 and 33 milligrams of caffeine per 8-ounce cup of decaffeinated coffee, depending on the brand of the coffee shop (a cup of regular has between 145 and 272 milligrams).

Until more studies are forthcoming, I would err on the side of caution and classify all coffee, black and green tea, chocolate, and cola drinks as caffeine-containing. And with caffeine, less is better. According to Dr. John F. Greden, a psychiatrist at the University of Michigan, large amounts of caffeine can cause a syndrome called "caffeinism," which is suspiciously similar to an anxiety attack: nervousness, anxiety, irritability, muscle twitching, jitteriness, and insomnia. Studies have shown that five or more cups of coffee per day seem to exacerbate cardiac trouble. Caffeine stimulates the adrenal system, the fight-or-flight mechanism that is associated with adrenaline. For this reason, it does make us alert, but it also accelerates the heart rate and constricts the blood vessels, raising blood pressure. When they stop using any amount of caffeine, even as little as one cup of coffee daily, most people get withdrawal symptoms such as headaches and fatigue, which usually disappear in two to seven days. Therefore, caffeine use is best tapered off gradually. It's also important to be careful with over-the-counter headache remedies: many of them contain caffeine, thereby stopping the symptoms but prolonging the addiction.

The amount of caffeine needed for adverse effects depends on the individual. Habitual coffee drinkers may be more used to the drug and need more to notice reactions than those who habitually drink little or none. I don't drink coffee at all. Still, some caffeine gets itself into my system on occasion. I also found myself at one point with occasional skipped heartbeats or brief flutterings. Then I decided to clear all the caffeine out of my body—no more black tea, green tea, or *anything* with chocolate. It took a few days of adjustment, and lots of extra sleep, but that was the end of my irregular heartbeats. I wonder how many people who end up on heart drugs and pacemakers could be cured by totally eliminating caffeine from their lives.

Alcohol

The abuse of alcoholic drinks (wine, beer, and hard liquor) is one of the risk factors for osteoporotic fractures and a number of studies show that alcoholism decreases bone formation, especially in men. The good news is that, according to a study at the Research Unit of Alcohol Diseases of the University of Helsinki in Finland, this problem is reversed within two weeks after complete abstention. With life's habitual pendulum swing, in the case of postmenopausal women the reverse may be true: researchers with the Framingham Heart Study, a forty-year-long ongoing study of heart disease and its risk in the residents of Framingham, Massachusetts, concluded in their 1988–89 evaluation that alcohol intake of about 7 ounces per week appears to be associated with higher bone density in postmenopausal women, possibly because alcohol augments the body's estrogen levels. (On the other hand, it might also increase hot flashes! Sorry about that.)

Alcohol abuse is frequently associated with magnesium deficiency; this in turn can cause a lower production of parathyroid hormone and so interfere with mineral absorption. In some cases, people who drink too much may ignore food and so lose weight; this weight loss also presents an increased risk for hip fractures. Some people are able to drink prodigious quantities of alcoholic beverages and show little in the form of "drunkenness." I particularly remember an older couple, friends of mine, who habitually had cocktails by 11 A.M. and continued from there; they never came across as "drunk." This may be convenient, but it is not necessarily an indication of health. The opposite, in fact, may be true. "Every drop of alcohol burned in the tissues creates a nutritional demand for carbohydrates and for the many biochemicals that it does not by itself supply, the vitamins and minerals necessary to process it," wrote George Watson in his classic book *Nutrition and Your Mind.* "One's tolerance to alcohol reflects the state of one's nutritional biochemical health. The more one can drink without adverse effect the worse off one is." For those who show the effects, the instability of gait and incorrect distance judgment that come with excessive drinking can cause falls, which may result in fractures if the bones are already thin.

On the whole, most studies point out the dangers of excessive alcohol intake. For those who insist on drinking, moderation means no more than one drink a day for women and two per day for men. Common sense says that it pays to be safe by using this drug within such limits.

Nightshades

The concept that the nightshade vegetables affect calcium balance has been put forth, for over twenty years, by Dr. Norman Childers, a professor of botany at the University of Florida at Gainesville and formerly of horticulture at Rutgers University. The nightshades are a botanical classification of plants, a family named Solanaceae; a subgroup, or genus, is called *Solanum*. This group comprises about seventeen hundred different plants. Some plants in this group are poisonous or medicinal, such as deadly nightshade, belladonna, and mandrake. Included among these plants are

Potato
Tomato
Eggplant
Peppers (red, green, hot, sweet, chile, paprika, jalapeño, poblano, etc., but not white or black pepper)
Tobacco

Professor Childers has shown that nightshade consumption correlates with osteoarthritis, because these plants contain substances called "alkaloids" that disturb the calcium metabolism, and tend to remove calcium from the bones causing aches, pains, even deformations. Dr. Childers has found that when people with arthritis, joint pain, bursitis, and bone spurs stop using these foods, their pain and symptoms abate dramatically after four to six months.

It has been my speculation since the early 1980s that people eat so many nightshades simply to counterbalance their consumption of milk products, which have more calcium than human beings need. For example, per 100 grams, mother's milk contains 33 milligrams of calcium, while cow's milk contains 118 milligrams. If we assume that the milk from each species is perfectly tailored to the needs of its young, it makes sense that cow's milk has four times more calcium than human milk. After all, it's designed to help a calf grow its bones up to cow size—not what a human needs! The calcium in cow's milk, then, is excessive for humans. How do we handle this excess? What I've noticed is that in a dietary system high in dairy, people commonly also eat plenty of nightshades: pizza, eggplant parmigiana, potatoes and sour cream, curries and yogurt, and so on. I believe that the nightshades might help in breaking up or neutralizing the excess calcium.

Theoretically, then, dairy and nightshades are opposite and complementary: if you eat one, you need the other. Conversely, if you stop eating one (say, dairy) you might do well abandoning the other, or else there may be repercussions in the body's calcium balance. Some people are very good at balancing milk products and nightshades, and do not seem to react to either, remaining free of arthritis, joint pains, bone spurs, or other calcium problems. Others are highly sensitive to these plants, and feel pains in their joints as soon as they eat even a little. Many of my students and acquaintances have found that if they keep eating nightshades in a low-fat, dairy-free diet, their joints begin to ache. The "growing pains" in children and teenagers may be associated with their extensive consumption of the tomato and potato nightshades.

Fortunately, the aches and pains will reverse in four to six months if the nightshades are removed from the diet. For those who really love them and want to eat them anyway, I suggest looking at what Greeks and Italians have traditionally done for generations: use the nightshades with plenty of olive oil and small amounts of feta or Parmesan cheese. While I have no actual data on the effectiveness of this suggestion other than the traditional usage, it seems to work very well with the taste buds.

I haven't found any studies that directly link osteoporosis and nightshades. Nevertheless, it may be sensible to pay attention to them because of their ability to affect calcium balance. For those at risk for osteoporosis, an occasional potato or tomato may not cause any trouble; however, it may be a good idea to refrain from relying heavily on these vegetables in the diet. In all cases in which I inquired, women with osteoporosis and a history of bone fractures relied on heavy daily use of potatoes as a major source of starch, and tomatoes as both a flavoring and a raw vegetable. One woman who took a number of classes with me and wasn't particularly bothered by her high-nightshade diet found herself with considerable thinning of the bones before she reached sixty. Rather than using potatoes as a major source of starch, it would be better to use whole grains such as barley, kasha, brown rice, and quinoa. Instead of using tomatoes or hot peppers to flavor everything, a better choice would be aromatic herbs such as oregano, tarragon, marjoram, and the like.

Citrus Juices and Vinegar

While above I mentioned that fruits are alkalizing, because of their potassium content, which is also the case with extracted juices, the latter nevertheless may contribute to mineral loss. Citrus fruits are rich in nutrients, as all natural fruits are. Juices, on the other hand, are missing the solids, and with that, the important nutrients that balance those in the juice; therefore, drinking the juice may create a relative condition of imbalance. While I've been saying this for years, as an intuitively obvious point, I reiterated it in an interview with *Self* magazine in July 1995. The author of the article, Diane Di Costanzo, didn't take my word for it and had the pulp analyzed. She wrote that "An analysis of 100 grams of orange pulp discarded from a juice extractor proves Colbin's point: the discarded pulp contains 6 percent of the oranges' vitamin C; 72 percent of the calcium; *all* the folic acid; and 76 percent of the fiber." Emphasizing the importance of these findings, she continues "It's the fiber that may help prevent some cancers as well as stave off energy swings. Fruit juices deliver sugars to the blood like a bullet, creating a spike, followed by a crash. Fiber slows the absorption rate of sugar to the blood."

This high amount of sugar, plus the natural acids, which you can recognize by the level of sourness in the taste of the juice, could *in some conditions* affect the body's mineral balance. The same is true for vinegar. The conditions in which this effect could happen are, in my observation, long-term low-fat diets, both omnivorous as well as vegetarian, as well as low-fat dairy-free diets. Note that the discarded pulp also contains 72 percent of the orange's calcium content! Clearly, it's better to eat the whole orange.

Weight Loss and Low-Fat Diets

One of the major risk factors for osteoporosis is being too thin. For women especially, this is a problem. Our current fashion dictates that "you can never be too thin" (or too rich, but that is another issue). Unfortunately, in terms of health that is not true: you *can* be too thin, as in gaunt, emaciated, and starved, particularly if over fifty. Malnutrition is possible, even in our society of abundance and excess, simply as a result of poor food choices. In terms of bone health, this condition can mean that if noticeably thin, both men and women are at risk for fractures, particularly when older. Women need between 22 and 27 percent body fat, says ob-gyn

Christiane Northrup; top models and anorexics may have as little as 10 to 12 percent, which is not enough for hormone production.

People can be too thin from different causes. In our culture, excessive thinness is mostly the result of some type of food restriction, either because of careless, nonnutritious eating, or purposely for weight control, for health, or for spiritual or political reasons. Strict calorie restriction, anorexia, unbalanced or inappropriate vegetarian diets, and junk food diets high in refined carbohydrates (white flour and sugar) all can bring it on. (Some diseases, such as cancer and AIDS, can also cause excessive thinness or wasting; however, these problems are beyond the scope of this book.)

Most women put on weight after menopause, much to their chagrin, from the same foods they used to eat for years without any weight problem. Their metabolism can change to such an extent that even fasting or dieting can actually increase their weight! Rather than fighting nature, let's look at what is going on, because nature has its reasons and reason cannot always second-guess it.

Once the ovaries stop producing estrogen, a woman's body keeps on making small amounts of it from subcutaneous fat, especially abdominal fat. Therefore, the extra weight is actually a good thing for menopausal women, believe it or not! Putting on this weight will help protect the bones, not just because of the continued natural estrogen production, but also because the strain of carrying the extra weight is a form of exercise and makes the bones work harder against gravity, thus helping to preserve bone density.

Obesity is known to be protective against osteoporosis; perversely, it is also a risk factor for heart disease and diabetes and does require a change to a healthier diet. At the very least, people with excess weight would do well to increase the amount of fruits and fresh vegetables in their diet to reach five to seven servings daily. An extremely restricted diet after menopause that keeps the body as thin as that of a teenager could cause problems. In fact, weight loss is a known risk factor. According to the National Institute on Aging, women who lose 10 percent or more of their body weight after the age of fifty have twice the risk of breaking a hip than women who don't lose weight. This is an extremely difficult notion for women to accept, as we hear over and over again that we should in fact return to our girlish figures. Impossible! And not even desirable. I think that older women who are excessively thin rarely look as good as thin young girls. A little plumpness may just fill in the wrinkles and actually make them look better. My school friend Elida, after hitting menopause, commented, "At this stage of the game, it's either your face or your butt. I'll take the face anytime!"

Weight loss by fat restriction appears to directly cause bone density loss; therefore, extremely low-fat diets can increase the risk of osteoporosis. In addition, vitamin D, necessary for the absorption of calcium from the intestines, is a fat-soluble vitamin. It is possible, then, that a long-term, chronic deficiency of healthy fats in the diet can contribute to bone thinning because the body can't absorb and retain the necessary calcium for lack of this vitamin. In his book *Nutrition and Physical Degeneration*, Weston Price mentions the story of a young boy with a leg fracture that hadn't healed in three months; the boy, who had almost constant seizures, subsisted mostly on white bread and skim milk. Dr. Price put him on whole wheat gruel made from freshly ground wheat, whole milk, and a teaspoon of special high-vitamin butter with each meal. Within a month the fracture had healed, his convulsions disappeared, and within six weeks he was running and jumping over fences like any normal boy. Dr. Price also found that household pets that are given white bread, sweets, and jams develop malformations of the bones and jaws.

Lack of Exercise

The bones are designed to function in opposition to gravity and movement. If we deny ourselves that movement, if we mostly sit, ride, take elevators, and avoid walking as much as possible, the bones will feel useless and perhaps just decide to fade away. Sometimes immobility is unavoidable, as in cases of serious illness when the sick person is bedridden or unable to move. Bone loss is then an inevitable side effect of that condition.

Children are often prevented from walking and running by constantly being required to sit down "and be quiet," in carriages, in car seats, in buses, in schools; these habits of restricted motion may carry over into adulthood and help create the proverbial "couch potato." Jean Liedloff, in her magnificent book *The Continuum Concept*, points out that children between birth and about age one are meant to be carried upright, in arms or in a sling, and participate in the movement of the mother's body, instead of being laid down in carriages and cribs. She contends that the absence of that period of being carried, what she calls the "in-arms phase," has lifelong implications. While I am not in favor of children running around in restaurants or at dinnertime, it could very well be that their hyperactivity at inappropriate times sometimes may be an outlet for the many hours of being still or sitting that our social system asks of them.

Intense Athletics and Excessive Exercise

Life is so perverse. Or perhaps we should say it is inevitably and always a seesaw, a Ping-Pong game, a pendulum swing. Trouble always arises at the extremes. Consider the following facts:

- Lack of exercise or movement causes bone loss.
- Exercise such as walking and weight training promotes healthy bone.
- Too much exercise or high-intensity athletics causes bone loss.

While these statements appear contradictory, they're all true; I'm not making them up. Studies have shown over and over again that female athletes, especially when their body fat is very low, at about 10 to 12 percent, lose their periods because their estrogen production is diminished by the lack of body fat. This lack of estrogen in turn causes bone loss. But it's not just the women, and not just the estrogen. A study of a college division male 1-A basketball team found that bone mineral content (BMC) decreased 3.8 percent from preseason to midseason, increased 1.1 percent during the off-season, and decreased another 3.3 percent during summer months when practice sessions resumed.

Once again, too little is no good, and too much is no good either.

Pharmacological Drugs

Our drug culture is pervasive and widespread and permeates every aspect of our lives. And I'm not talking about recreational, illegal, or street drugs; those are just the shadow side of the main drugs of our society, the ones sold by prescription or over the counter in numerous legitimate establishments. Several of them directly affect the health of our bones.

Steroid Drugs

These drugs, also called corticosteroids (cortisone, glucocortisone, glucocorticosteroids, and others of similar names), are used fairly widely in pill, inhalant, or cream form against all kinds of inflammation and skin irritation, as well as arthritis and asthma. They can damage the bones because they interfere with the absorption of calcium from the small intestine into the blood. Bone thinning and osteoporosis can result from this interference, sometimes very quickly. A 1993 study published in the *Annals of Internal Medicine* found that steroids can cause an 8 percent reduction in bone mass (which is the same as what happens with removal of the ovaries), within four months of use. In Great Britain, a poll of fifteen thousand users and former users of the drugs found that fully 50 percent had developed osteoporosis. Bone loss from the forearm, for example, can go as high as 10 percent per year in adult subjects taking corticosteroids; as contrast, the normal loss from this site is between 0.5 and 1.5 percent per year after the age of fifty.

Steroids are dangerous drugs and have well established, serious adverse effects; these include weight gain, bruising, pain in the back and legs, cataracts, diabetes, muscle weakness, mood swings, and the well-known "moon face." However, if you are taking steroids and are questioning their role in your bone health, under no circumstance should you just stop taking them: suddenly discontinuing the use of these drugs can be very dangerous, and only an experienced physician should monitor their gradual withdrawal if and when it is warranted.

Antacids

These over-the-counter, nonprescription drugs are widely used for digestive distress. Their purpose is to *anta*gonize the *acids* in the stomach, which supposedly contribute to the discomfort felt by many people after eating. A little thought will illuminate what an insane notion that is. Stomach acids are essential for digestion; if the stomach is uncomfortable, why target its natural process? Why not change the input, so that the natural acids can work properly? Here, as elsewhere, I think of Dean Black's comment in his book *Health at the Crossroads*: "Nature has its own laws, and does not tolerate intrusion without revenge."

If digestion is uncomfortable, then the practical and sensible things to do if we want to solve the problem would be chewing the food thoroughly, changing the diet, and drinking enough water (as opposed to soft drinks). But that's not what most people do, thanks to the relentless advertising, nor is it even what doctors recommend. The treatment of choice is usually based on various over-the-counter or prescribed pharmaceutical drugs.

Antacids neutralize acids by adding alkalizing substances to the stomach. These drugs are based either on aluminum hydroxide or calcium carbonate. Regarding the former, considering the concern with aluminum in the brain of people with Alzheimer's disease, it always comes as a surprise to me that little is said about the aluminum in these and other commonly available OTC drugs. Aluminum hydroxide antacids have been associated with bone pain and multiple stress fractures. Calcium-based antacids have become extremely popular as a calcium supplement to ward off osteoporosis.

There are a number of scientific papers describing the unexpected problems that a large, unbalanced influx of calcium has on the human body. Excessive calcium intake may inhibit the absorption of iron and zinc. One of the bigger problems is severe kidney failure necessitating hospitalization and even dialysis. The condition caused by excess calcium carbonate is called *hypercalcemia* or *milk-alkali syndrome* (see page 21), which can be life-threatening if not caught in time. The symptoms include reduction in physical fitness, fatigue, headache, nausea without vomiting, abnormal bone scan, abnormal parathyroid hormone levels, and kidney failure. Medical students have an easy way to memorize the problems associated with this condition: "Moans, groans, bones, and stones."

With the increased use of these antacids as nutritional supplements, hospital admissions for hypercalcemia went from less than 2 percent before 1990 to more than 12 percent between 1990 and 1993, according to a study published in the journal *Medicine* in 1995. The condition is reversible if caught early enough and treated appropriately; in some cases, however, residual kidney damage may remain.

People often take antacids habitually and regularly for years. I once saw a man for a consultation who had been taking a popular aluminum-based antacid for ten years, twice daily, and he had developed ALS, or Lou Gehrig's disease; I strongly felt that there was a connection between the two. A study in Germany described a man who had been taking a calcium-based antacid daily for more than four years to deal with stomach pains; his CAT scan showed calcifications of the kidneys, which improved somewhat but not totally after treatment.

What other effects could antacids have if they're taken for another purpose, such as in the attempt to prevent osteoporosis? It would seem to me that they will still interfere with the digestion process; as there is no indigestion, the interference is unnecessary. As a result, I imagine that there could be some type of malabsorption, nutrient deficiency, or the like. And how will this show up? My guess is that there will be digestive discomfort and a general feeling that things aren't right. If that is not attended to, other manifestations of digestive interference may appear, but I don't know what they might be. If you are taking antacids for calcium, and you "don't feel quite right," consider that there might be a connection.

Warning Signs

The body is a rational entity, once we understand how to translate its communications to us. It will not go from perfect health to major illness in a day. Generally there is a slow buildup, or breakdown if you wish, with little complaints and minor symptoms that, on the whole, we either ignore or suppress with drugs. Here I'll focus on the small warnings our body gives us when there is trouble with the bony system deep within, so that we can take appropriate measures to forestall worse trouble.

Basically, the warning system associated with osteoporosis relates to the structure of the body in general, and to the body's mineral and protein stores. What follows is a list of areas to note that are associated with these nutrients, and where deficiencies may show up first.

Bad Taste in Mouth upon Arising

My personal observation is that when we eat acid-forming foods (flour, sweets, protein) without enough alkalizing soups and vegetables, there is a strange, sticky-sour taste in the mouth when we wake up, as well as a whitish coating of the tongue. It may be accompanied by bad breath as well. I always consider this an alarm symptom, because it indicates to me a condition of acidosis, which will eventually draw calcium out of the bones so as to neutralize the excess acids in the blood. Please note that it is almost impossible to test for this, as the metabolic buffering process takes place within minutes.

Most people will try to fix the bad taste with juice, coffee (both alkalizers), and of course brushing the teeth. However, getting rid of the taste is only half the job. If you are familiar with this bad "morning mouth," experiment with changing your diet. I believe the best way is to wake up with *no* taste in the mouth, and that can be done through careful dietary choices, such as more alkalizing soups (try vegetable and miso soups), foods, drinks; less baked and fried flour-based foods, less fatty protein foods, more vegetables, and eliminating desserts.

Hair and Nails

Both hair and nails are extensions of the skin, composed mostly of protein. They contain no nerves and therefore have no feeling; however, they are not "dead," but very much alive and constantly growing. At their point of original growth—the hair bulb and the nail fold and bed—they are nourished by the blood, so they can easily show the condition of the body's nutrient stores. In severe cases of malnutrition, for example, the hair becomes brittle and can be pulled out with no pain. Alternating periods of protein-energy malnutrition and good protein intake can result in a condition known as "flag sign," where the hair loses and then regains its pigmentation resulting in alternating bands of pigmented and white hair.

Dry, dull, brittle hair and weak, thin, peeling nails can be a sign of insufficient protein intake, a condition that can result from diets with a high proportion of carbohydrates such as flour, bread, pasta, grains, and sugar, a low proportion of fats and protein, or generally too low in calories. As bones need protein for their flexibility, a long-term protein and/or calorie deficiency that has been signaled through hair and nail weakness can eventually lead to brittle bones, regardless of the intake of calcium.

Teeth and Gums

The wisdom of the body determines that imbalances will show up first in areas of least survival value, and then progressively go deeper. In addition, Chinese medicine as well as other systems of diagnosis consider that the outside is always a reflection of the inside, so that trouble inside the body generally shows up with some external manifestation. As the jaws are part of the skeletal system, and teeth need minerals as much as bones do, trouble with the teeth and gums can then be an indication of impending or current trouble with the bones. A study published in the *International Journal of Prosthodontics* in 1996 found that women with osteoporosis have significantly higher gum recession and therefore are at higher risk of losing their teeth than people with normal bones. Another study, this one in *Age and Ageing*, found that a decrease in bone density in men was consistently associated with increased tooth loss. Postmenopausal women with osteoporosis also have a higher than expected number of dentures, as well as fewer teeth than women without osteoporosis.

Before we get to tooth loss and advanced gum disease, we get other signals. In my own experience, I found that certain foods seem to have some effect on teeth, and so possibly on the skeleton in the long run. For example, sour foods such as vinegar, citrus, and tomatoes, when eaten in a low-fat, low-protein diet, can damage the enamel or even cause toothaches. The toothaches are usually in teeth already weakened by cavities, even when filled. In my own case, I found that once when I had orange juice (freshly squeezed!) every day for a month, one of my wisdom teeth (the one with the big cavity) started hurting quite acutely. My dentist had no solution other than to offer to yank the tooth, which I was not ready to do. So I tried to get rid of the pain by following a rather "politically incorrect" diet for a few weeks: no fruit, no salad, no vinegar, no juices, and plenty of butter and olive oil on everything. I even ate a few good portions of brie! It worked within a week. Once the pain was gone, I cut down on the fats, was able to eat fruit again sporadically, and salads as usual with modest amounts of dressing. I'm not sure how this worked, but it did; I had simply followed my instincts in eating what *felt* right at the time.

Joints and Back

Aches and pains are a warning symptom from the body that something needs to be attended to. Taking painkillers to get rid of the pain is not only dumb, it's disrespectful to our bodies. Would you cover up the dashboard of your car if its lights go on because your brake fluid is low? Of course the problem often is that we don't have a good model to help us figure out *why* there is pain, *what* it is saying, and *what to do about it*. If a light went on in the dashboard and it had no explanation, you would probably ignore it or cover it up for lack of knowledge. Let me then give you a few pointers that I have found to be very helpful in diminishing or eliminating minor aches and pains.

If they are in the muscles or the joints, there are three things I look at, foodwise:

- Intake of raw foods, fruits, and juices, sodas, and alcohol *in a low-fat diet*
- Intake of nightshade vegetables (tomatoes, potatoes, eggplants, and all the peppers, as detailed earlier)
- High intake of calcium and vitamin D in supplement form

When any of these three is noticeable in the diet, I would correct it in the following way. For the first one, either eliminate them completely, *or* drastically increase your intake of *healthy* fats. Perhaps both, depending on how much your joints hurt. For the second one, definitely eliminate them all for a few months. Yes, it takes that long sometimes to have results, because the body needs to rebuild itself. For the third one, I would eliminate the supplements entirely and rely more on nutrient-rich foods. In addition, check your condition with a doctor, good chiropractor, and/or acupuncturist, to make sure there is no serious damage.

For pain in the back, I would first of all go to a good chiropractor or osteopath. If nothing shows up there, a good deep tissue or shiatsu massage can be helpful in loosening tight back muscles. Low back pain, incidentally, has been considered to be a risk factor or warning signal for osteoporosis. Heed the warning, change your diet, do more walking, stretching, and gentle yoga, and look at whatever other areas of your life give you pain. Just make sure to face the issue and not deny it, then you can avoid making it worse.

Stress

When we are under constant pressure, always meeting deadlines and fighting the competition, our adrenal glands, the secretors of the fight-or-flight hormone adrenaline, go into overdrive and eventually into exhaustion. Lack of protein and excess carbohydrate fuel this process further. Dr. Christiane Northrup points out that women with high rates of cortisol hormones in their saliva as a result of stress are the most apt to get osteoporosis.

Other Alarm Symptoms

Linda Ojeda, in her book *Menopause Without Medicine*, lists, in addition to the above, other alarm symptoms that may signal osteoporosis well before the bones break.

Among them are

- loss of height (which may indicate collapsing vertebrae)
- nocturnal leg cramps
- transparent skin
- rheumatoid arthritis
- restless behavior (food jiggling, hair twisting)
- insomnia

All these are indications of lack of calcium or magnesium in the body. Should you find yourself with any of these symptoms, review your diet, your activity level, the medications you take, and the amount of coffee and alcohol you consume. It may be time to check with a health professional or nutritionist, and develop new health habits.

Dwelling on Our Weaknesses

If our bones are our structure, keeping us upright, they relate metaphorically to our psychological and spiritual structure. If we look at the body as an expression of our inner selves, perhaps of how we think of ourselves, what would make this structure weaken over time?

When we are young, in our teens and early twenties, most of us feel invincible. Death will never get us. We can do anything. We know better how things should be done than all those so-called adults. And then time goes on, and we begin to find our limits, discover our weaknesses, and, eventually, feel that death is coming closer. Perhaps a weakness in our bones shows us our fear, our lack of connection with a core sense of self, of reality. Perhaps it shows us that we lack a support system we can fully rely on.

Women are subject to fear because of the relentless social communication that tells us that, once we reach menopause, we're not good enough. We are suffering from "hormone deficiency," even though we are perfectly in tune with the natural order that is set up to diminish our hormones. We are "putting on too much weight," even though the natural order causes such weight gain for evolutionary reasons, to protect, in fact, our bones. We are "getting too wrinkled," we are no longer "sex objects" for every man (although we may in fact have happy and fulfilling sex lives with our individual partners!), and old women have no respectable place in our society. All these messages go to the deepest core of our self-esteem. Our mothers may have felt the same insecurities, and passed them on to us. Therefore, we feel that if we don't take the hormones, lose the weight, cream or cut our wrinkles away, try to look "sexy," and attempt to keep the place we had when we were younger, then we have utterly failed at being women. We fear that we have failed at "aging gracefully" anytime we don't look younger than we are. What an impossible situation.

If we are living in fear, with no good role models of strong older women, with a destroyed sense of self-value, ignored or shunted aside by society, the media, even at times our children, we weaken and collapse figuratively. And so do our bones, literally.

What Weakens Bones

Acid-alkaline balance: Acid-forming foods (protein and carbohydrates) drain calcium from the bones; alkalizing foods (fruits, vegetables, seaweeds) neutralize the acids and prevent calcium drain.

Calcium-mineral drainers: acid-forming foods, caffeine, alcohol, nightshades, citrus juices and vinegar

Other factors that weaken bone: weight loss, lack of exercise, excessive exercise, pharmacological drugs (steroids, antacids)

Alarm symptoms: bad taste in mouth on arising; trouble with hair, nails, teeth, gums, joints, or back; loss of height; nocturnal leg cramps; transparent skin; rheumatoid arthritis; restless behavior (food jiggling, hair twisting); insomnia

---

Now that we have the bad news, let's look at the good news and see how much we can do for ourselves in strengthening our bones.

5

What Strengthens Our Bones: The Conventional Approach

It is frightening how dependent on drugs we are all becoming, and how easy it is for doctors to prescribe them as the universal panacea for our ills.
  —Charles, Prince of Wales, 1985 address at 150th
  anniversary dinner of the
  British Medical Association

What We Are Told

The relentless bombardment of advice on how to prevent osteoporosis includes the following:

- Get plenty of calcium: drink milk, take supplements.
- Take a bone density test to see how you're doing.
- Take hormone replacements if you're a menopausal woman.
- Take drugs to keep the bones from remodeling.
- Exercise.

Do these recommendations work? Does our population have fewer bone fractures if they are followed? Well, Jane Brody, the well-known *New York Times* medical reporter, in one of her 1997 "Personal Health" columns discussed her friend Helen, who "was certain that osteoporosis was one problem she would not have to worry about. She had been taking estrogen since menopause and calcium supplements for years. She quit smoking decades ago and remained unusually physically active throughout her adult life." Already in her 70s, Helen regularly walked for exercise, cycled, played tennis, and ice-skated daily all winter. And yet one day, on the rink, she collapsed with a broken hip and arm, without having tripped or slipped. In other words, her bones broke simply from gravity, rather than from trauma. Unfortunately, the reporter goes on to assume that the problem occurred because Helen had not been taking other drugs to slow down the loss of bone. I would say that what Helen's unfortunate condition shows is that the current recommended regime is not working, and adding more drugs to the mix is unlikely to make things better. In fact, I wonder whether the current regime of hormone replacement and calcium may not be making the problem worse, perhaps in some ways that we have not yet discovered.

With the recommendation for exercise I have no quarrel. However, because of my observations and experiences, I do not believe that preventing or treating osteoporosis with drugs, pills, and milk products is the right way to go, and Helen's case proves my point. After all, one of the most interesting epidemiological aspects of the condition is that it occurs more in cities than in rural areas. Therefore, coincidentally or not, those people who have more access to drugs and pharmacies also tend to have more osteoporosis than those who still rely mostly on traditional and folk healing systems—what we now call "alternative" or "complementary" medicine. Whether there is a causal connection remains to be established, but I believe the coincidence is meaningful. Let's take a brief look at the other side of milk products, supplements, hormone replacement therapy, and pharmacological drugs that affect osteoporosis. After that, we'll look at what you can do naturally to strengthen your bones.

A word about bone density tests: Research shows that higher bone density does not necessarily indicate a lower risk for fracture. In fact, one woman who came to see me for a consultation had been told she had high bone density, yet she had broken her wrist twice within a year. These tests, the most common of which is "dual energy X-ray absorptiometry," are being widely touted and prescribed. Susan M. Ott, an associate professor at the Division of Metabolism at the University of Washington in Seattle, has been warning for some years that there is insufficient data to predict whether the relative risk of fracture changes with a change in bone mass. In a 1994 editorial in the *British Medical Journal* she points out that there can be numerous problems with these tests due to the imprecision of instruments, errors in interpretation, and other technical errors. In other words, a single test means relatively little. In addition, Dr. Ott says that the incidence of fracture doubles every decade on the same test reading, so fracture risk has a lot more to do with age than with test results. The World Health Organization has decreed a "normal" bone density arbitrarily, rather than by studying the median value of healthy subjects and then coming up with the numbers; by doing so the organization has placed a lot of asymptomatic, healthy people (mostly women) in the "abnormal" range. I have seen no comments on the risks of radiation exposure through bone X-ray tests, by the way. .

Lorna Sass, Ph.D., the author of many cookbooks such as *Cooking under Pressure* and *The New Soy Cookbook*, is suspicious. "I am beginning to feel there is something not quite trustworthy about these tests," she told me. "*Everyone* who gets tested is told they're not normal for their age. Then they're told to take drugs or hormones." Not only that, but the pressure is intense: the endocrinologist who reviewed Lorna's test told her that her bones would fracture by the age of sixty or sooner if she didn't take hormones or bisphosphonates. Physician Christiane Northup points out that for small-boned women, the test may suggest that the bones are brittle and at risk, even when they aren't. Lorna is very small boned.

Perhaps the most important thing to do is to look at all the risk factors. Anything a test can tell should be supported by other information. When there are two or more risk factors such as malnutrition, a high proportion of processed foods and refined carbohydrate consumption, lack of vegetables or protein in the diet, steroid or other drug use, excessive thinness, alcoholism, advanced age, and sedentary living, the test could then have more validity.

What About Milk Products?

It is common knowledge that milk products are a source of calcium, thanks to the relentless marketing of the dairy industry. They are also high in protein. In fact, the lower the fat, as in skim and fat-free milk products, the higher the protein. For example, while a cup of whole milk has 8.03 grams of protein (and 4% fat, by the way), a cup of low-fat (2%) milk has 8.12 grams, and a cup of skim milk (0%) has 8.35 grams.

The problem with milk products is that many people find them mucus-producing, and allergies to these foods are extremely common. Colds and ear infections in children who are taken off milk, cheese, and ice cream often diminish or disappear. The consumption of milk products is associated with numerous health problems in women, including chronic vaginal discharges, acne, menstrual cramps, fibroids, chronic intestinal upsets, and benign breast conditions, as pointed out by Dr. Christiane Northrup in her book *Women's Bodies, Women's Wisdom*. Eliminating dairy foods improves all these problems, as well as endometriosis pain, allergies, sinusitis, and recurrent yeast infections. Nursing mothers who consume a lot of milk products may provoke colic or cow's milk allergy in their babies; some studies also find a correlation with juvenile diabetes and milk intake. Let's remember a simple concept: milk normally goes out of the woman, it should not go in. When it goes in, it goes the wrong way.

While milk products are a natural and traditional food, in most traditional societies they are not part of the native diet. Therefore, most people in the world lose the activity of the lactase enzyme that digests lactose, and become what is known as "lactose intolerant." This is in fact not a disease, but the normal state of adult mammals, the species to which we belong. Societies that continue using milk products into adulthood, such as the Northern Europeans, are only 2 percent lactose intolerant, while other societies that do not consume them, such as the Malays and Filipino, are as much as 98 percent lactose intolerant. The condition manifests as digestive disorders, stomachaches, bloating, gas, and diarrhea with the consumption of milk products.

For all of these reasons, I do not generally consider dairy products a good-quality calcium source. Instead, we can get our calcium from the same place where the cows, the horses, and the elephants get theirs: green vegetables. And if you're thinking "Well, I (or my kids) just don't like vegetables," that is precisely the issue: if you eat milk products you *naturally* don't like vegetables. Why not? Because milk is just vegetables that went through the cow. Your body knows you've already had them. Why should you have them twice? Both adults and children who don't consume milk products like vegetables just fine.

If you are in a situation where there are few or no vegetables available, no seaweed, no parsley, no soups or stocks, then milk products would be necessary as a source of calcium, provided you are not allergic to them. If you decide to continue using caffeine or nightshades, a small amount of dairy is also appropriate. Among milk products, the most healthful are natural, full-fat whole milk (without added synthetic vitamin D), whole milk cheese, and yogurt from organically-raised, hormone- and antibiotic-free cows. Cultured and fermented milk products are the easiest to assimilate. On the other hand, skim or fat-free milk and cheese would be proportionately too high in protein, thus increasing the acid load and contributing to calcium loss. The natural butterfat, together with the calcium, buffers the acids; it also helps absorb the protein better. There is a reason why nature puts all these nutrients together, and we are fools to think our technology can do a superior job in making this product healthier.

In the face of the propaganda pushing milk as a good source of calcium and therefore a preventative of osteoporosis, let's remember that osteoporosis is more common in dairy-consuming countries such as Northern Europe, Canada, and the United States. Not only that: An article in the June 1997 issue of the *American Journal of Public Health* found that, in a study of seventy-eight thousand nurses over twelve years, women who drank two or more glasses of milk a day were more likely to fracture a hip or forearm than those who drank milk only once a week or less. In other words, "purposeful behavior itself is often counterproductive" when we look at only a small part of the picture (calcium in this case) and lose sight of the whole (the context of milk drinking). If we remember that a bone high in calcium but low in the protein matrix is more likely to fracture, it seems to me that the admonition to keep piling up the calcium (out of context) could in fact be totally counterproductive.

Be especially attentive to how milk products affect the rest of your health, including allergies, colds, mucus conditions, skin outbreaks, digestive disorders, and overweight. Because I have seen so many people who got rid of those conditions when they eliminated milk products, I believe that on the whole most people are better off without using them regularly. For that reason, you will find almost none in the recipe section, except for butter, ghee, and a little Parmesan. If you like to consume milk products more regularly, or use them in your cooking, make sure that they are from healthy cows fed healthy foods, unpasteurized, not homogenized, and with no added vitamins. Organic butter from cows that graze on green grass is naturally high in vitamins A and D, and therefore appropriate as a condiment when available.

Pills and Drugs

The medical model we live by relies greatly on man-made substances to maintain or enhance our health. These substances are usually presented in pill form, but are also available in the form of syrups, drops, and injections. I maintain that it is entirely possible to be healthy without having to take pills of any kind, especially those that are either self-prescribed or suggested as "why don't you try this?" (Obviously, medications that are lifesaving are a different story.) For osteoporosis in particular, numerous medications, supplements, and drugs are regularly recommended as prevention. It is well known that *all* man-made drugs or supplements have unbalancing or adverse effects. It's even more serious when more than one drug is taken, as often there is not enough information as to what they do when they interact within the body. For men and women over seventy, in fact, combining drugs may cause real problems: one study in Rouen, France, found that 15 percent of patients had experienced drug-interaction side effects, some of which were serious enough to require hospitalization. Using drugs to prevent something that may *or may not* happen could cause adverse effects that may be worse than the problem presumably avoided. It is advisable to assess carefully the risks of taking these drugs before taking them.

Considering how clear it is that these substances are a double-edged sword, I am mystified by the enormous appeal of pills and drugs. Perhaps it is because they seem so magical: "Take this pill, and you'll get better without any effort on your part!" But magic has its price. Sometimes we find out that the price is much more than what we were willing to pay—as in the fen/phen fiasco, where the price of possible weight loss turned out to be an irreversibly damaged heart.

The Issue of Supplements

We know that foods are made up of nutrients—vitamins, minerals, protein, fats, carbohydrates—and that we need an optimal amount of them in order to be healthy. Nature has set up the system by which these nutrients are delivered in the best and most accessible form: they come in packages, in certain proportions to each other, in the foods we eat. These are fruits, nuts, leaves, roots, tubers, and vegetables such as broccoli and cauliflower; the foods derived from animals such as meats, fish, fowl, eggs; and the foods resulting from agriculture such as whole grains and beans. Milk products have only been used traditionally by a few populations such as the Swiss, the Laplanders, and the Hindi.

Things changed when food processing was discovered. White flour was made by sifting out the bran and the germ; the resulting flour was shunned by insects and rodents, a detail that should have given us pause. What happened instead is that the forces of commerce found value in the "shelf life," and adopted this devitalized food as the base of breads and cakes. Abundant amounts of fats and sugars had to be added to white flour to make it palatable. Even pasta made with white flour needs plenty of sauce to make it palatable; in fact, sauce is the *only* thing that makes a pasta dish memorable. Try eating pasta with nothing, and you'll see what I mean: it's empty food.

Sugar—white cane sugar—is another element completely stripped of any nutritional value. The original cane has, as nature ordained, plenty of fiber and minerals; getting the sweetness out of five or ten inches of sugar-cane could keep one occupied all day long. But to get one cup of crystalline white sugar, one needs seventeen feet of sugarcane. What a waste! How much nutrition is thrown out with all that cane fiber?

After a few decades of consuming refined flour and sugar in the nineteenth century, vitamins were discovered, and by the early twentieth century most of them had been found and named. Soon they were being extracted and sold separately. I remember in the fifties there was so much excitement about concentrating the "active ingredients" out of foods, that there was talk of a "lunch pill." We wouldn't have to bother with eating anymore!

Well, the lunch pill never made it to the stores. There is more to food than the nutrients we can chemically extract from them. Flavor, aroma, texture, crunch, and that certain feeling of having enjoyed a good meal— none of that is available with the lunch pill. Not to forget, of course, that there probably are nutrients in foods that we haven't discovered yet.

On the other hand, individual nutrients do have a medicinal value, demonstrated in numerous scientific studies. Vitamin C definitely helps heal scurvy, a disease common in those who eat no fruits or vegetables, subsisting instead on white bread, meat, and alcohol; B vitamin supplements have helped overcome beriberi and pellagra, which appears when people subsist on polished white rice or degermed cornmeal. These are just two very old examples where individual vitamins help overcome the deficiencies of a refined-foods diet devoid of fruits and vegetables. Numerous studies as well as popular books point out the many different benefits of individual nutrients for a vast array of conditions. This information has then been extrapolated into the idea that taking multiple vitamins is essential to good health, and is now firmly established. Unfortunately, this is not always the case, as we shall see.

The ability to digest and absorb food varies from person to person. Among the causes for malabsorption of nutrients are

- years of eating processed and refined foods,
- diseases of the small intestine, and
- the use of antibiotics, which destroy the intestinal flora.

Processed and refined foods can, over time, leave undigested residues along the digestive tract that eventually prevent the absorption of many nutrients. Diseases of the small intestine, such as celiac disease or sprue (the inability to tolerate gluten), frequently result in the malabsorption of vitamin D and minerals. Antibiotics damage the intestinal flora responsible for the synthesis of B vitamins and other nutrients, and thereby weaken or destroy the ability of the bowel to absorb them. In these cases, careful and *individualized* nutrient supplementation may be in order. In other words, each person's nutritional supplementation regimen must be prescribed, after a thorough health history and appropriate tests, by a trained health practitioner. Self-prescription of drugs or supplements is inadvisable. We can cause as much damage from having too much as we can from having too little.

One of the drawbacks of supplementation is that it bypasses the body's natural efforts to draw nutrients out of food, and therefore creates an atrophy of sorts. If we get used to natural foods that have the nutrients hidden in the cells, our digestive system becomes quite adept at pulling them out and absorbing them. On the other hand, if we continuously feed our bodies with already preabsorbed or readily available nutrients in pill form, one or two things may happen: the body becomes lazy and loses the ability to absorb nutrients from food, thereby becoming more and more deficient even in the presence of nutritious foods, and/or the body does not absorb the nutrients and they pass right through, wasting both money and energy.

One of my students told me about her parents, who regularly take their supplements, and who at one point had to drain the cesspool of their house. The workers found a ten-inch layer of pills on the bottom of it!

On a spiritual level, taking supplements without real medical need is based on the emotion of fear, particularly the fear of not having enough. If fear is the motivating factor, perhaps it would be more effective to address that deep-seated feeling than douse ourselves with pills. I prefer to trust that there will be enough of what we need for all of us. Let's remember that in going for the apparent benefit in a straight line, we may once again be "generating unending secondary consequences" and causing ourselves unexpected troubles. Taking calcium supplements is a case in point.

Calcium is the main recommended nutrient to prevent and slow down osteoporosis. But do we really need it in pill form? Leo Lutwak, M.D., in his book *The Strong Bones Diet* (with Lois Goulder), points out that many women who take daily calcium supplement pills may develop abdominal discomfort, constipation, or even kidney stones, and not know there is a relationship. Excess vitamin D, often found in calcium supplements, if more than 1,000 IU per day, may provoke bone loss. "There are advantages to getting your calcium from foods instead of pills," Dr. Lutwak writes. "Bone health depends not only on calcium, but on many other nutrients that are contained in different kinds of foods."

As Lutwak and Goulder point out:

- Foods high in calcium also contain numerous other vitamins and minerals.
- Vegetables high in calcium are fine sources of fiber, which prevents colon cancer and contributes to satiety as well.
- Foods provide energy, pills don't.
- While you may forget to take your pills, you will generally remember to eat.

There is much more uncertainty about taking calcium supplements, that seemingly universal recommendation, than one would suspect.

How Much Calcium?

In the United States, the Recommended Daily Allowance is 800 to 1,200 milligrams (mg) per day. However, the World Health Organization recommends only 450 mg per day; at that level, people in Third World countries do not have the high rate of fractures found in more developed countries. In the United States and United Kingdom, 26 percent of the female population show osteoporosis, and they have vertebral crush fractures by age sixty-five; of these women, 35 to 40 percent have at least one hip fracture by age ninety. In South Africa, rural Bantu women have one-tenth of the hip fractures of Caucasian women; yet they consume only half the calcium (250 to 400 mg), even into their ninth decade. They bear on average six children and breast-feed them for two years. White women bear two children and feed them formula diets. Why is there such a discrepancy?

The reason may be found in the rest of the diet. Context counts. In June 1994, the Consensus Development Conference on Optimal Calcium Intake, sponsored by the National Institutes of Health, recommended as much as 1,500 mg for women over fifty who are not taking estrogen. However, in the same conference, Dr. Robert P. Heaney, of Creighton University in Omaha, pointed out that the amount of sodium and protein in the diet are crucial variables for the amount of calcium needed. When the diet is low in sodium and protein, the daily calcium requirement for an adult female may be no higher than 450 mg, the amount recommended by the WHO and easy to reach on a diet based on beans, grains, and vegetables, with small amounts of animal foods and fats, which is what most traditional people in the world eat. This is the system on which the recipes of this book are based. On the other hand, if the intake of sodium and protein is high, as in a commercial or junk food diet, a woman may need up to 2,000 mg to maintain the calcium balance between nutrients.

That, at least, is the current theory. In 1987, the NIH Conference on Osteoporosis found that barely 13 percent of cases could be attributed to low calcium intake. The Nurses Study by D. Feskanich, Walter Willett, Meir Stampfer and others at Harvard found that a dietary calcium intake higher than 450 mg per day *doubled* the risk of hip fracture, and that was on a standard American diet. What is more interesting to me is that the high calcium intake was obtained by drinking milk; that is, women who drank two or more glasses of milk per day had a 50 percent higher risk of breaking a hip than women who drank less than one glass per week. In the typical understatement of scientific writing, the authors state that "the data do not support the hypothesis that higher consumption of milk or other food sources of calcium by adult women protects against hip or forearm fractures." A 1997 study by Cumming, published in the *American Journal of Epidemiology*, found that the use of calcium supplements was also associated with a doubling of the risk of hip fractures, and the use of a popular brand of calcium antacids brought a 70 percent increased risk of forearm fractures.

Excess calcium—out of its natural context, that is, in supplement form—can cause other problems. The mineral is involved in muscle contraction, which is important for the continued regular beating of the heart. Therefore, too much of it can cause the abnormal heart rhythms and chest pains of heart disease, which is then often treated with a type of drug called *calcium channel blockers*. According to Ruth Winter, a medical writer and author of many books, calcium-based medications may cause stomach bleeding, nausea, vomiting, excessive thirst, or abdominal pain, and should be used with extreme caution by people with heart or kidney disease.

I would say that any factor that doubles the risk of fractures ought to be considered a serious problem, and people should be warned against it; unfortunately, our social marketing system is quite far from turning against the use of milk products and calcium supplements as preventors of osteoporosis. It also took some time for people to figure out that the world wasn't flat.

Nature protects us from excess and imbalance by always building checks and balances into foods. As we saw in chapter 2, an excess of calcium creates a relative deficiency of magnesium, and may create symptoms associated with those deficiencies. We also need magnesium and vitamin D to absorb calcium properly. The point then is to consume calcium *within its natural context*, together with the other minerals and vitamins that the natural order has placed nearby. That is how our bodies are programmed to absorb and utilize all nutrients. Whenever we take one nutrient out of context and consume large amounts of it, all other nutrients then become relatively insufficient.

Alendronate or Bisphosphonates

Often I get the impression that in our search for health we tend to look for the miracle cure, the magic "bullet" or, rather, the magic pill. This search prompts us to explore different options in conventional Western medicine just as much as it may lead us to the so-called alternative modalities. Drug medicine is extremely effective at finding substances that manipulate and maneuver the body to do one thing or another; unfortunately, we know that drugs usually have a backlash because they tamper with a natural order that their promoters consistently ignore.

So now we have the magic of alendronate, also known generically as bisphosphonate (I've omitted their brand names, which often change). Alendronate is prescribed to increase bone density and prevent bone loss; it does so by interfering with the process of bone resorption, that is, it stops the bone from releasing calcium and minerals into the bloodstream. Rather like putting a freeze on your calcium bank withdrawals. Deposits are OK, withdrawals are stopped; ergo, bigger bank accounts, bigger bones. The drug seems to increase bone density and decrease the risk of fracture by more than 40 percent.

As always, there are adverse or side effects to these drugs, which have caused many a user to stop taking them. They appear to cause serious burning in the esophagus, a type of heartburn, which does not respond to antacids. These effects may be lessened if they are taken with a glass of water on an empty stomach, without taking anything else and remaining upright, maybe walking or riding a bicycle for thirty minutes. I've spoken to a number of women who couldn't continue taking these drugs because of the side effects. Others had no problem.

But if we have here a type of drug that seems to provide a measurable health benefit, knowing that to every action there is a reaction, I have two big questions: If you cannot withdraw your money from the bank, eventually you will run into problems with the landlord and the phone company, to say the least. If you cannot withdraw calcium from your bones to handle the needs of your heart, muscles, and nerves, how is that deficiency going to show up later? How long will it take? Will we be able to correlate, say, muscle tremor with the use of these drugs, and not have it be ascribed to coincidence or some other "disease"? And if this drug burns the esophagus to such an extent when it is taken, what else will it burn as it moves through the body?

As Professor Susan Ott points out, while the drugs increase bone density in postmenopausal women by about 5 to 10 percent over one year, after

t the density appears to plateau, because bone formation stops if resorp-
on is halted, so no new bone is made. In addition, "the long-term effects
of interfering with the remodeling cycle are still not known. Subtle side effects may be those on the bone itself. These might go undetected, since
bone pain or fractures usually are attributable to the underlying disease" or
osteoporosis.

At the time of this writing, the drug has been tested for a little over three
years. Many women are now taking it, unwittingly taking part in something
called "postmarketing surveillance." That is, the users of the drug will be
monitored, either formally or informally, to see what other good or nasty effects could come from it. That means that users of this relatively new drug
are, knowingly or unknowingly, participating in a large trial. On top of it,
they (or their insurance company) will have to pay to be part of it. Not all
users will suffer from the unknown or unexpected side effects of this drug.
Not all actual adverse effects will be accurately ascribed to it. Different body
types will have different adverse effects. How will we ever know? In the
meantime, I would watch out for cramps of any kind, as well as an increased
risk of heart attacks, both of which can be related to low blood calcium.
Time will tell. Most serious side effects of drugs are not noticed for almost
twenty years, or perhaps a whole generation (more than twenty-five years).

Estrogen Therapy

It is true, and we saw it in chapter 2: female hormones do promote the
deposition of bone matter. As estrogen wanes with menopause, this particular bone stimulator becomes less prominent. If we do nothing else, and
if on top of it we eat mostly acid-forming foods such as sugar, coffee, meat,
pasta, bread, and potatoes, our bones will indeed become thinner. But is
the answer really in putting back what nature removes? What are the "unending secondary consequences," or, as they are generally known, the "side
effects" of this particular practice?

Estimations and interpretations vary. It is generally accepted that the
risk of breast and endometrial cancer is higher in women who take hormone replacement therapy (HRT). According to Carol Rinzler, author of
Estrogen and Breast Cancer, the studies that have found an association between estrogen and breast cancer consistently find a 30 to 40 percent increased risk of the disease in women who take the medication. Other risks
include venous thromboembolism (VTE) or deep vein blood clots, gallstones and gallbladder disease that may require gallbladder removal, and
the inconvenience of breakthrough bleeding in postmenopausal women.

While hormone therapy may result in a temporary slowdown in bone loss, after it is stopped bone loss accelerates to "catch up" with the normal rate. For example, women who took HRT for ten years after menopause and then stopped would have lost 27 percent of their initial bone density by age eighty, while those who were never treated would show a loss of 30 percent. As most hip fractures occur after the age of seventy-five, HRT does not appear to be a good preventative measure, unless it is taken for the rest of one's life and one is willing to risk the other problems it may bring.

Risks of Hormone Therapy

- Increased risk of endometrial cancer
- PMS symptoms (swelling, bloating, breast tenderness, mood swings, headaches)
- Menstrual discharge
- Increased risk of breast cancer
- Stimulation of the growth of uterine fibroids and endometriosis
- Increased risk of gallstones and blood clots
- Possible weight gain

Source: C. Runowitz, M.D., "Hormone Therapy: When and for How Long?" *HealthNews,* March 25, 1997

Using sex hormones to affect the function of bone seems a bit far-fetched. Professor John A. Kanis, of the University of Sheffield Medical School in Great Britain, published a study in the November 1996 issue of *Bone* where he questioned the logic of "targeting women at risk from osteoporosis at the time of the menopause when the benefits and risks of HRT are largely *extraskeletal*" (my emphasis).

In one of those perverse twists that life's pendulum swing often brings, a study published in the *Journal of the American Medical Association* in 1996 found that women with denser bones have a 2.0 to 2.5 times higher chance of developing breast cancer than women with lower bone mineral density. The authors of the study called for identifying a common denominator for these conditions. However, as pointed out by Lynne McTaggart of the newsletter *What Doctors Don't Tell You*, they neglected to factor in the use of HRT, which is known to increase bone mass and also to increase the risk of breast cancer. Why do the women in this study have higher bone mass? It could be because of exercise, good diet, or, not improbably, the use of

HRT. Surely the authors of the study should have known that particular variable. As HRT both increases the risk of breast cancer and thickens the bones, we now have a Robin Hood situation: synthetic hormones take away from immunity so as to give to the skeleton.

Hormone replacement therapy has been sold to women by tapping into their fear of aging, a modern fear embedded into our consciousness by the youth culture. It is foolishness to try to "reverse aging." There is nothing wrong with aging itself. As we get older, there are many mistakes we don't have to make again, many insecurities we can give up, many dangers we can laugh away. And aging does not invariably mean illness and broken bones; there are plenty of older people in their seventies and eighties who are in fine shape and excellent spirits. Of the people I know who are in their seventies and eighties, those that are the healthiest are those who are the most physically and mentally active. Broken bones are not the result of "estrogen deficiency": *all* women have lower estrogen levels after menopause, but only 25 to 30 percent of them get fractures. These are more often than not the result of our lifestyle choices, overall weakness, ill health, or prescription drugs.

We may also want to consider the symbolic and spiritual aspect of taking female hormones. What is the background emotion? Surely it's obvious to us all. Fear rears its unpleasant head again, the fear of not being the approved image, not being attractive, desirable, sexy, "feminine"—the fear of getting older, heavier, slower, an image that is never presented in our media as a desirable role model or a valid stage in a woman's life. Add to that the fact that most grandparents don't live near their grandchildren, that many older people live in secluded communities, and that therefore the image of aging is far away and hidden from us. How much we lose when we lose that part of life! The images I grew up with, on the other hand, from my mother and other European relatives, friends, and acquaintances, is that older women looked so good, were so together, knew how to handle life so well, that I was actually quite impatient to get to being "older." I don't think I felt that I was quite old enough until after I turned fifty, in fact.

According to Carol Ellis, M.D., a New York City general practitioner, the long-term use of hormone therapy is still somewhat controversial among physicians. There may be on occasion valid medical reasons for its use, perhaps temporarily, to treat such conditions as *severe* hot flashes or sleep disturbances. Considering their attendant cancer risk, to use these powerful drugs as a preventative for bone loss is questionable to say the least, considering how many other, less dangerous options we have.

Strengthening Bone: Conventional Suggestions

Milk products are not appropriate for many people, either because of allergy or sensitivity. In addition, they are no guarantee against bone fractures, as there are more of these in countries that consume dairy than in those that don't.

Drugs and pills: Supplements, hormone replacement, and other drugs always have a backlash adverse effect; best used only with extreme caution in advanced cases.

There are better ways in which we can strengthen our bones and keep them strong. Let's now look at the more natural approach that I propose.

6

Strengthening Our Bones: The Natural Approach

Where illness takes the shrivelling form leafy vegetables are in order.
— Rudolph Hauschka, D.Sc., *Nutrition*

Good Food

In the natural order, we can get all our necessary nutrients, in the correct proportion, from the foods that nature provides. Every traditional society before the invasion of the Europeans had well-balanced, abundant, and nutritious foods on which they lived for many generations. For example, at the archaeological site of Ceren, in El Salvador, a village from about A.D. 560 preserved in volcanic ash, there is evidence of abundant food such as corn, several kinds of beans, squash, chile peppers, avocados, nuts, and fruits. Animal proteins were obtained from deer, ducks, dogs, and freshwater mollusks. As archaeologist Payson Sheets, from the University of Colorado at Boulder, commented, "The standard of living fourteen hundred years ago was higher than it is now."

In our civilized modern times, food quality is not nearly as good as it has been for thousands of years. Three factors contribute to this problem:

Poor soil: The land has been overfarmed by monoculture, and the soil is damaged through the use of artificial fertilizers, pesticides, and herbicides, often petroleum-derived.
Poor food quality: The majority of the foods promoted to the public are refined, stripped of their natural nutrients, canned, frozen, artificially colored, artificially flavored, and otherwise doctored with thousands of different chemicals.

Poor health: Many people are unable to absorb fully the nutrients from the food, mostly because of problems in the digestive tract.

These three factors are behind the tremendous increase in the popularity of nutritional supplementation. While it can be—and has been—very successful in many cases, let's always remember that all man-made or extracted substances invariably have adverse as well as beneficial effects. Not everything can be treated with a vitamin pill. Here are better ways to counterbalance the above three factors:

Choose organically grown or raised foods. These are grown without artificial fertilizers or pesticides, in soil that has been free of these chemicals for at least three years. Organically or naturally raised animal foods are not treated with antibiotics or growth hormones, and are given natural feed. These are generally available in farmers' markets and natural food stores, but more and more supermarkets are carrying them as well. Just ask.

Choose only fresh, natural, unrefined foods. These are available in all markets as well as in many natural food stores. That means we need to pick foods that have to be prepared from scratch: whole grains and whole-grain breads, beans, fresh vegetables, fruits, nuts, seeds, organic eggs, fish, organic or free-range fowl, and so on.

Prepare and eat your foods with care and attention. People with absorption problems need to cook their food well to make it more easily digestible. Raw vegetables and salads may be hard for them to digest because of the excessive roughage; in that case they would be better off with soups and stews. Fruit is easily digested for some people, too gas-producing for others. Most important: chew your food thoroughly.

Foods to Emphasize

For an optimum intake of minerals, nothing beats *fresh vegetables, organically grown.* Include in your diet five to ten servings daily from a variety of:

- Dark leafy greens, both cooked and raw: kale, collards, mustard greens, turnip tops, watercress, arugula, chicory, escarole, spring greens or mesclun salad, fresh chopped parsley, and the like

- Carrots, parsnips, yams, turnips, rutabaga or yellow turnips
- Cruciferous vegetables such as broccoli, cabbage, cauliflower, Brussels sprouts
- All other vegetables, including onions, celery, garlic, ginger, radishes, and scallions
- Beans, which are a good source of cholesterol-free protein as well as calcium

Another excellent source of minerals is the use of *homemade stocks*, made with bones or vegetable scraps.

Protein is essential for giving bones the flexibility that prevents fractures. There is controversy as to which kind is better, animal or vegetable. We've heard that a diet high in animal protein can contribute to osteoporosis. On the other hand, in one study on mice, not only did the animal protein diet result in bones more resistant to breakage than did the plant protein diet, but the animals fed animal protein were seemingly less affected by variations in intake of phosphorus and calcium than were the animals fed plant protein. My viewpoint has always been that this choice is a very personal one, and that either one can support good health, as long as the issues of quality (freshness, lack of food additives, naturally raised without antibiotics or hormones) are addressed. For *protein foods*, include two or three servings daily of either

- Fish, organically raised fowl or meat, organic eggs
- Beans: lentils, split peas, kidney beans, navy beans, black beans, and the like
- Nuts and seeds: sunflower or pumpkin seeds, almonds, cashews, walnuts
- Sesame seeds, which are also high in calcium and essential fatty acids

Soy foods are a fine protein food for people who are not allergic or sensitive to them. In addition, they contain certain substances that are estrogenic, and help in lowering the incidence of hot flashes and other menopausal symptoms. I do not recommend such highly processed soy products as texturized vegetable protein (TVP). You can include in your diet, two or three times weekly, the most traditional soy products, such as tofu, unpasteurized miso, and tempeh. Some studies show that certain phytoestrogens in soy foods slow or stop bone loss.

Several women of my acquaintance found that just drinking a glass of soy milk a day helped eliminate their hot flashes! However, I don't recommend soy milk as a regular drink for everyone. Soybeans contain thyroid-lowering factors (known as "goitrogens") and too much of them could interfere with the body's natural thyroid function.

If you include these foods in your diet, you'd do well to follow the example of the Japanese and also include high-iodine *sea vegetables* in your diet, which nourish your thyroid and counterbalance the soy. They are also high in many other minerals, such as calcium, iron, phosphorus, magnesium, and zinc. Have them two or three times weekly, and choose among nori, hiziki, arame, kombu, dulse, kelp, or alaria.

For *fiber*, the best natural source of all the *B vitamins*, and the most balanced source of complex *carbohydrates*, include two or three servings daily of whole grains: brown rice, barley, buckwheat or kasha, millet, quinoa, cornmeal, oats, and whole wheat (if you're not allergic to it).

Thomas Cowan, M.D., suggests that millet is best for older people, as it is rich in silica which helps keep the bones supple. Remember that when consuming whole grains as well as any other starches, it is essential to *chew each bite thirty to thirty-five times*! For proper digestion, the salivary amylase enzyme, or ptyalin, needs to reach all the starch molecules to start the breakdown process, which will then be completed by the pancreatic amylase enzymes in the upper part of the small intestine. When people don't chew their grains properly, they may experience gas or bloating or abdominal discomfort two or three hours after eating.

For the best of health, it is important to eat food cooked from scratch, rather than with the use of canned and frozen ingredients. These may be convenient, but they lack "prana" or "chi," that undefinable life energy that replenishes us and gives us zest. Freshly prepared, home-cooked meals are absolutely essential to our well being.

Specific Dietary Influences

What we eat is really a major influence to help create and maintain strong bones. As we saw earlier, focusing only on calcium is not going to be enough. We have to look at the total diet, and at the relationships and interplay of all nutrients.

In chapter 4 we looked at the foods that tend to *drain* calcium and other minerals from the bones, thus *promoting bone resorption*. Now we'll look at which foods increase the mineral load of the body to encourage or *promote bone deposition*. Throughout, let's keep in mind that foods can act in opposite ways depending on their excess, their deficiency, or their relationship with other foods and nutrients. For example, excess protein (usually animal protein) may cause calcium loss in the urine and perhaps contribute to osteoporosis. On the other hand, a lack of protein would weaken the collagen matrix of the bones and so also contribute to osteoporosis. Nice conundrum, isn't it?

Calcium-Mineral Boosters

Many foods will contribute calcium, magnesium, and other minerals essential for continuous healthy bone formation. The main categories are plant foods, stocks and bones, and good-quality fats. Let's take a look at them.

Plant Foods

Calcium and other minerals are found abundantly in the vegetable kingdom, especially if organically grown. Of particular interest are all the green leafy vegetables, such as kale, collards, mustard greens, arugula, bok choy, parsley, watercress, as well as broccoli, cabbage, carrots, and acorn or butternut squash. Interesting note: The food that provides the most calcium *per calorie* is bok choy, at 790 milligrams (mg) per 100 calories, cooked. Other leafy greens range from 164 (broccoli) to 250 (raw celery) to 495 mg (cooked mustard greens). As a comparison, skim milk provides 351 mg of calcium per 100 calories.

Some vegetables such as spinach and Swiss chard, in addition to containing calcium, also contain substances called *oxalates*, which may interfere with calcium absorption in some cases. However, people on low-calcium diets (300 to 400 mg per day) are more efficient at overriding the effect of oxalates and absorbing calcium than people on diets high in calcium-rich dairy products.

Sea vegetables, or seaweeds, are one of the best sources of minerals. These are common foods in other parts of the world such as Japan and Ireland; however, in our society they are not part of the usual pantry. Most commonly, people eat sea vegetables in Japanese restaurants when consuming "miso soup," "sushi," or "nori rolls." In the natural food world, these foods are also popular, especially with those who follow a macrobiotic-type diet.

Even though sea vegetables are uncommon, it pays to use even a few of them in stocks and condiments as suggested further on in the recipe section. A study of osteoporosis in Taiwan found that those who include seaweed in their diet two or more times per week showed a slightly higher protection against osteoporosis. These foods are extremely rich in calcium, magnesium, phosphorus, manganese, boron, and more than thirty other minerals; because they are so rich, a little goes a long way. Of particular interest is the fact that they are a good source of iodine, necessary for healthy thyroid function, which also influences bone health. However, for those who consume iodized commercial salt, seaweeds would offer much too much extra iodine; one of the two should be avoided, and I suggest avoiding iodized salt and just getting the mineral from the natural source of seafoods and sea vegetables. I found it very interesting in my classes that often people with diagnosed low thyroid function invariably love seaweed!

Dry beans and peas are an excellent and often overlooked source of both calcium and protein. Nuts and seeds also are fine sources of both, in addition to providing vitamin E and essential fatty acids.

Stocks and Bones

While the muscle and organs of animals are very poor sources of calcium, bones are obviously an excellent source of all bone-building minerals. They are not, however, easily edible. How to get at their valuable nutrients? There are several ways.

First of all, stocks made with animal bones or seafood shells can be a very important calcium source. Adding a little bit of vinegar or wine to the stock while it simmers will drain calcium from the bones or shells, and make it available in the stock. See the recipe section for a variety of fish, chicken, beef, and vegetarian stocks; make big batches, freeze them, and use them in all your cooking, especially to make soups and whole-grain dishes.

Another way to get at the calcium in the bones is to eat them whenever they are edible. Canned salmon, often recommended as a source of calcium, is such only when the soft, well-cooked bones are consumed as well. Sometimes people eat the salmon meat and throw away the bones! Fresh small fish with bones, such as sardines, smelts, and whitebait, are also a good source. However, the disadvantage with these is that for the bones to be edible the fish is usually prepared by deep-frying. While the high heat softens the bones and makes them edible, at the same time the heated oils create trans fatty acids that could in the long run contribute to cancer and aging, so fried small fish are best used very sparingly. I found, however, that a very satisfactory way of preparing these foods is by tossing them with a little olive oil and then baking them; you'll find the details in the recipe section, together with their incredibly high calcium content. Roasted chicken, if well done, often has the wing tips and drumstick ends softened, so they can be munched on; some people really like to chew on all the bones for a while, which is an excellent idea. Good for the teeth, too.

Cooking fish or chicken on the bone helps increase the mineral content of your meal: during the cooking process, a little of the calcium will migrate into the meaty part, so even if the bones are not consumed at least there will be small amounts available in the edible part.

Healthful Fats: Why They Are Important

Fats have been getting an incredible beating in the past few years. They have practically been considered equivalent to evil poison; many otherwise sane people avoid fat as if it were a direct insult. So much fear and loathing are unwarranted. Fats are one of the three essential macronutrients that provide us with calories. As a concentrated source of energy, fat is essential in cold climates as its breakdown provides us with heat. A layer of fat under the skin insulates the body from environmental chills and helps keep it at a steady temperature. This same layer of fat (perhaps a bit thicker) can produce estrogens, and so helps women in menopause and beyond keep their hormone levels up naturally. The kidneys, heart, and liver need to be surrounded by fat deposits so as to be protected and held in place.

Good-quality fats, in small amounts, are needed for the proper function of the immune and hormonal systems, the manufacture of prostaglandins, sex hormones, cell wall construction, and the transport of fat-soluble vitamins such as A, E, K, and D. Udo Erasmus, author of *Fats that Heal, Fats that Kill*, says that essential fatty acids are closely involved in the metabolism of calcium. One of the more obvious connections is the fact that vitamin D is fat soluble, and if we are fat deficient, we will also be lacking in that vitamin, which in turn will affect our absorption of calcium.

As Erasmus points out, some fats heal, some fats kill. The unhealthful fats are refined, heated, or hydrogenated. They are found in fried foods, commercially processed products, and animals raised on poor diets, drugs, and no exercise.

Among the worst sources of fats are chips and snacks, crisp baked goods (always a sign of high saturated fat presence, often in the form of margarine or shortenings), candies, and commercial milk products, especially commercial ice cream (because of its high sugar content). The unhealthful fats contribute to cardiovascular disease, obesity, diabetes, immune system dysfunction, cancer, and osteoporosis. As they slow down the digestive process

---

Unhealthful Fats

- Refined oils (corn, safflower, soy, canola, etc.), all fats with no taste and no flavor
- Hydrogenated fats such as margarine and shortening, because they're high in trans fatty acids
- Any fat heated above the temperature of boiling water, or about 200°F.
- Animal fats from cows, pigs, and chickens raised with agribusiness methods
- Whole milk, butter, cream, yogurt, ice cream, and cheese from cows raised on antibiotics, hormones, and junk cow food instead of plain grass and water

---

by cutting down the secretion of hydrochloric acid in the stomach, these fats contribute to slow digestion, indigestion, and poor absorption of nutrients.

One modern risk that we are a long way from assessing is the use of genetically engineered foods. Canola oil, which is a refined fat but very popular as a purported source of omega-3 fatty acids, could be made from genetically engineered seeds. The process of genetic engineering is subject to error as all man-made things are. According to *Rachel's Environment and Health Weekly #549*, a quantity of canola seeds enough to seed between 600,000 and 750,000 acres of land was recalled in Canada in April 1997 because the specific gene used in the crop had not been the type approved for human use. What is really scary is that no one, except the parent company, could have known the difference. There was a well-publicized 1988 case in which the genetically engineered amino acid L-tryptophan had unexpected trace contaminants that caused a painful disease called eosinophilia-myalgia syndrome (EMS) that affected almost ten thousand people and killed thirty-seven. What else could happen to our immune systems when they are exposed to more and more foods "improved" by these newfangled technologies?

Nature does the job right. Healthful fats are high in essential fatty acids (EFAs), which include omega-3 and omega-6, both associated with cardiovascular health, good skin, lustrous hair, good nails, and a strong immune system. When they are unrefined, they contain their natural antioxidants and nutrients. Mostly they are found in nuts, seeds, and fresh cold-water fish such as salmon and mackerel. If chickens and cows are raised on natural foods and no drugs, they have a higher proportion of monounsaturated fats and lower cholesterol. EFAs prevent calcium from being excreted in the urine. Good-quality saturated fats are also necessary for important metabolic functions, according to Sally Fallon and Mary G. Enig, Ph.D., because they

- constitute at least 50 percent of cell membranes,
- help in assimilating the EFAs,
- protect the liver from alcohol ingestion,
- enhance the immune system,
- have antimicrobial properties and, most importantly,
- play a vital role in bone modeling.

The saturated fats protect the calcium-depositing mechanism in bones from free radical disruption. (Free radicals are those highly reactive molecules that are involved in essential energy production throughout the body; some of them [between 2 and 5 percent, according to Udo Erasmus] may cause damage to tissues and cells, and are neutralized by antioxidant nutrients such as vitamins C, E, carotene, and bioflavonoids.) Fallon and Enig further point out that populations in tropical areas, where the saturated coconut and palm oils are regularly used in the diet, have very little osteoporosis. They also have little or no heart disease. According to Erasmus, we should note the fact that in the traditional tropical societies, the tropical fats they consume are usually fresh and unrefined, and so contain a number of additional nutrients such as carotene, vitamin E, and other components that contribute to the body's nutrient stores. These natural fats are a far cry from the bleached, refined, deodorized, hydrogenated oils and fats available in our stores, which are high in the heart-damaging *trans* fatty acids. For example, cholesterol supposedly is raised by saturated fats. However, a study in Malaysia, the world's major producer of palm oil, showed that this oil lowers cholesterol. Erasmus points out that the oil used in that study in all likelihood was fresher and more natural than that used in other studies in the United States.

I once had the opportunity to use fresh, unrefined palm oil from Africa. It was thickish and had a deep, rich orange color. When I used it for sautéing vegetables, I needed no herbs or other seasonings because the flavor was so wonderful, close to paprika yet without being a nightshade. There is no doubt in my mind that it was full of natural carotenes, and protective against damaging free radicals and probably good for the bones.

The omega-3 fatty acids can be found in fish, shellfish, fish oils, and flaxseed oil. The omega-6 fatty acids are found in meat and unrefined sesame, safflower, and sunflower oils. In Canada, the suggested omega-3 to omega-6 ratio is between 4:1 and 10:1. There is no minimum daily requirement established, but Udo Erasmus recommends that they comprise at least one-third of total fat consumed.

Healthful Fats

- Extra virgin olive oil
- Unrefined sesame and sunflower oil
- Cold-pressed flaxseed oil
- Traditional coconut and palm oils
- Butter or cream from healthy cows fed natural foods and no antibiotics or hormones (organically raised)
- The natural fats in eggs and animal foods that are organically raised or wild

---

Extremely high-fat diets can contribute to bone loss. For example, a very-high-fat diet (80 percent of calories), known as the *ketogenic diet*, has been used since the 1920s in a number of hospitals as a highly successful treatment for epileptic seizures, especially in children who do not respond well to antiepileptic drugs. Studies done on the additional effects of this diet have shown the following:

- At the beginning of its use, it creates metabolic acidosis, but the condition reverses itself within a few days even while continuing on the diet.
- Excretion of calcium in the urine was increased while calcium balance in the blood remained positive.
- One of the few observed adverse effects of the ketogenic diet was some bone loss.

The studies didn't point this out, but it seems to me that the calcium was removed from the bones to buffer the acidosis, which would explain all three findings. (Curiously enough, I found no evidence that the diet is correlated with an increase in heart disease.)

The ketogenic diet is obviously an extreme situation, as rarely will anyone go on an 80 percent fat diet by natural tendency. Yet on a standard American diet of processed and fast foods, snacks, dairy, and sweets, it is entirely possible to reach 40 percent or more of calories from fat, most of it in the form of unhealthful fats. This low-vegetable, high-unhealthful-fat, high-protein, high-refined-carbohydrate diet creates an increased tendency toward an acid condition, which in turn removes calcium from the bones, particularly when accompanied by lots of soft drinks and sweets.

So then the solution is to eliminate fats, right? Well, Mother Nature doesn't like to see anything eliminated. There is always another side of the coin. A *very-low-fat* diet will also hurt bone if

- it causes weight loss of 10 percent or more of normal weight
- it is an acid-forming diet high in flour, sweets, and/or protein and low in vegetables
- it is a diet high in nightshades and low in or devoid of milk products

With fat as with everything else, too much is no good, too little is no good. The average postmenopausal woman needs about 65 grams of total fat per day. Some dishes and some meals will have more and some less. That means we need approximately a total of two or three tablespoons of good-quality fat per day in an eating regimen that is based on home-cooked foods such as vegetables, beans, grains, nuts, and seeds; no more than one or two tablespoons of added fats per day when cooking with animal foods or dairy. Udo Erasmus cautions against using any one type of fat exclusively—e.g., flaxseed oil—because it might cause an imbalance in the fatty acids that it does not provide. A mixture of oils is best, such as extra virgin olive oil or unrefined light sesame and flaxseed oil, that can be used on salads and steamed vegetables. See chapter 8 for details.

The Role of Sodium

Sodium has gotten a bad reputation in the last fifteen years or so. This is unfortunate, as it is absolutely crucial to our health. It is an alkalizing mineral that is found abundantly in our bodies, especially in the fluids both outside (extracellular) and within (intracellular) all our cells, as well as in the bones. It works with potassium to balance the acid-alkaline factors in the bloodstream, and helps regulate water balance, muscle contraction, and nerve stimulation. It is essential for the proper function of our cells, nerves, and metabolism. Sodium keeps the other essential minerals dissolved in our blood, and so avoids the buildup of deposits. It helps purge carbon dioxide (which we breathe out) from the body and stimulates the production of hydrochloric acid in the stomach, thereby aiding digestion.

Sodium is found abundantly in nature and throughout our food supply, and not just in table salt, the basic NaCl or sodium chloride. It's in all natural foods such as meats, beans, and vegetables, in easily absorbable form. This is not really a problem. Where we run into trouble is with the sodium also found in many sodium-based ingredients, additives, and pre-servatives in commercial foods, such as bicarbonate of soda (baking soda), monosodium glutamate, sodium nitrite, and many others. Baked goods that contain baking soda and baking powder can be a highly significant, though often overlooked, source of sodium. Any ingredient with the word *sodium* or *soda* in it contains sodium salts. A quick look at a packaged food's ingredient list will tell you if there is sodium in it; the nutrition label will say how much.

Sodium-based Commercial Food Additives

sodium propionate	bicarbonate of soda
sodium stearoyl lactylate	sodium benzoate
sodium caseinate	sodium nitrate
sodium citrate	bicarbonate of soda
monosodium glutamate	sodium bisulfite
sodium nitrite	

The average appropriate sodium intake has been estimated by the National Research Council to be 2,300 mg per day, or about one teaspoon. While a necessary and essential mineral, a number of studies have shown that sodium will increase the urinary excretion of calcium, indicating bone loss, when consumed in excess (3,000 to 9,000 mg per day). A 1995 study on postmenopausal women at the University of Western Australia found that a reduction in bone loss, equivalent to the daily dietary *increase* of about 900 mg of calcium, can be achieved by simply halving the intake of sodium to about 1,200 mg per day.

There is a considerable difference between the traditional salt we get from drying up seawater, known as sea salt, that mined from old salt mines, and the pure, white, free-flowing substance from the supermarket. Commercial table salt contains a number of sodium-based additives such as sodium silico aluminate and yellow prussiate of soda, plus potassium iodide and additional additives of high cosmetic but questionable health value. Sea salt is the best salt to use in cooking, in modest amounts—that is, food should never taste salty, but the salt can be used just enough to brighten all the other flavors in the food. To keep the amount of sodium in your diet from being excessive, refrain from adding extra salt at the table.

Our concern for the excess sodium in our diets should be reserved mostly for processed foods. Plant-based foods such as celery contain sodium in addition to other minerals, but these are the beneficial natural sources that give us the sodium we need, and so pose no problem.

Water

While we think of water as a soft, fluid substance, it is in fact the strongest element on earth. Just think of this: Water can break rocks and glass, lift enormous weight in hydraulic lifts, and ravage everything in its path during a flood. It is the basis of all life on this planet. Recently there was great excitement about the possible discovery of water—or its traces—on Jupiter's moon, a discovery that could indicate the presence of life (at least of life as we know it).

Our human bodies are 60 to 70 percent water by weight. This water is within and around our cells, in our secretions, our blood, and our tissues. It travels freely throughout the body, passing through membranes and organs with equal ease. Even our bones contain about 22 percent water. According to F. Batmanghelidj, M.D., author of *Your Body's Many Cries for Water*, we may ignore, not recognize, or lose our sense of thirst, and thereby become mildy or chronically dehydrated. Among the symptoms of such dehydration are asthma, high blood pressure, diabetes, and pain in general, including stomach, angina, and joint pain, as well as low back pain, one of the indicators of possible osteoporosis. A sufficient intake of clean water is essential for the proper function of the entire body as well as the strength of the bones. About eight or ten glasses per day is the ideal.

Based on earlier studies I had undertaken, for a long time I disagreed with this viewpoint. Specifically, I thought that when one eats more whole grains, beans, and vegetables, one needs less water because there is so much water in the cooked grains and beans, and, of course, in the vegetables as well. Therefore, drinking much more than what one needs might overwork the kidneys. What I find now is that one has to look at the entire picture. The more dry or low-water foods one eats, the more water one needs. Dry or low-water foods are animal protein foods, baked flour products of any kind, nuts, and sweets. High-water products are fresh vegetables, fruits, and cooked whole grains and beans. Salty liquids, caffeine, alcohol, and sweetened drinks do not count as water because they are in fact diuretic.

How do we know if we've had enough water? The urine is on the light side, it is abundant, and one has to empty one's bladder about every two or three hours. More than that, and there could be either too much water, or some organic disorder such as kidney trouble or diabetes. Less than that, and if the urine is dark and scant, there is not enough water taken in and one can become dehydrated. Sometimes when people don't drink enough water during the day, they urinate little yet need to get up during the night to urinate. In these cases, drinking *more* during the day is the answer, so as to stimulate the kidneys to do their job during the daylight hours.

What kind of water? Much of our tap water has impurities or chemicals such as chlorine and fluoride. To eliminate the chlorine, it's enough to draw the water and then let it sit uncovered for a couple of hours so that the chlorine can evaporate. The fluoride, which is a by-product of steel manufacturing, is added to the water to keep children under the age of six from getting cavities, and therefore is a medication that may not be appropriate for adults.

It seems obvious to me that medicating the water is not a democratic idea; in addition to that, there are many health problems associated with fluoridation, such as an increase in uterine cancer mortality, a rate of dental fluorosis (fluoride-induced toxicity and tooth mottling) as high as 72 percent in children, lower fertility rates, and osteogenic sarcoma, a malignancy. A significant number of studies found that fluoridated water may in fact increase the rate of fractures, even though fluoride may provide a higher bone mass. For about thirty years, sodium fluoride was used as a treatment for osteoporosis precisely because of its ability to increase bone mass; as it was found that it didn't change the fracture rate, this treatment is generally no longer used.

To obtain the cleanest water possible, choose either a good filter, good-quality spring water in bottles, or fresh water from your own brook, spring, or well. Make sure to have the water tested for impurities, bacteria, and parasites. I do not recommend distilled water because it has been stripped of all life; it is quite akin to white sugar, and I maintain that it will draw minerals out of the body, and the bones, simply by osmotic pressure.

I find that room temperature water is best, rather than ice cold, because it is easier for the body to accept it and assimilate it rapidly. Normal body temperature is 98.6°F, and to bring forty-degree water up to that level takes the body a lot more time and effort than dealing with seventy-degree water.

Movement and Exercise

Now here is some information that probably is no news to most readers: exercise is good for the skeleton. Movement and weight-bearing exercises put stress on the long bones of the arms and legs, a factor essential to the continued process of bone deposition. When movement is lacking, as with sedentary or bedridden people, bones invariably lose mass. The influence of gravity is crucial: astronauts in space lost bone mass during weightlessness until they began doing special exercises to prevent this problem, stressing their muscles and bones against fixed points in the spacecraft cabin.

I'm so lazy that having to do exercise is a really boring activity for me, especially as it takes me away from reading or writing. However, after I got married in 1995 and saw myself on the video, I realized that the jig is up. If not for the bones, I'll do it for the flab. Vanity will get me going every time. So I've made a yearly New Year's resolution since then to do *something* regularly to get the old body moving, and I have pretty much kept it. I'm liking it, too, much to my surprise.

The body needs to move. Because of the way it is designed, walking is the movement that most efficiently puts just enough gentle strain on the bones to promote their continued re-formation. It also doesn't cost anything. Brisk walking or race walking are additional benefits; jogging and running, if the knees allow it, are more of the same but not essential. Swimming, while an excellent exercise, is not really weight bearing because it is the water, not the bones, that bear the weight. Water exercise, on the other hand, does count for bone health as it makes the body move against the resistance of the water. Golfing, as long as it promotes walking and not riding in a cart, is an excellent if high-priced way to protect your bones.

How does this work? When the heel hits the ground while walking, vibrations travel the length of the leg bones, and the stress creates a piezoelectric effect all along them, keeping the bone crystals together as well as attracting nutrients from the blood and encouraging them to be deposited onto the bone. Walking briskly on firm ground in shoes *with thin soles* is one simple way to encourage this process, and is in fact how human beings have been doing it for thousands of years. So what about those very thick rubber-soled sneakers? Perhaps thin-soled tennis shoes or light moccasins might be better. An article in the Tufts University *Health & Nutrition Letter* pointed out that athletic shoes with thick, spongy soles are the worst kind for maintaining balance and might lead to falls, especially in older people, because they don't allow for accurate perception about where your feet are in relation to the ground.

Breathing deeply, as most exercisers are apt to do, will indirectly protect the bones by reducing metabolic acidosis. Yoga and Tai Chi are excellent exercise systems for flexibility, balance, posture, and strength; they are generally gentle and easy, ideal for people of all ages. Tai Chi is practiced daily in China even by the elderly; you may have seen it on television or even in your local parks. I found yoga to be the most satisfying exercise as it just feels so good; it doesn't hurt the knees, and is generally credited with stimulating all the endocrine glands and lowering blood pressure to boot.

Training with light weights is excellent for bone strength. This is something you can do at home, and a set of weights is not very expensive. One study of postmenopausal women at the Veterans Administration Medical Center in Gainesville, Florida, found that weight training, by boosting the strength of legs, arms, and shoulders, increased bone density about 1.5 percent per year, while the sedentary control group actually lost about 2 percent. Over five or ten years, those numbers could spell a vastly lower risk for fractures. In addition, by improving posture and balance, all exercise will lower the risk of falls that may result in fractures. Not only that: A 1997 study by Dr. Laurence Kushi of the University of Minnesota School of Public Health, in Minneapolis, found that postmenopausal women who engaged in moderate activity (bowling, gardening, or long walks) four or more times a week were 33 percent less likely to die during the study than sedentary women.

Weight lifting, weight training, or just regularly lifting heavy things (such as big soup pots or buckets of water or toddlers) is very important for the continued buildup of bone. As women keep depositing bone to the age of thirty when they attain "peak bone mass," it seems to me that nature would take advantage of the fact that a woman might have had a good number of children by then and carried them about regularly. Therefore, it is really important for young women to do regular physical exercise and lift some type of weight so as to build good bone mass early in life. However, weight lifting works at any age. One study in a nursing home had sedentary older women start their exercise with soup cans—imagine being so weak from disuse that soup cans are heavy! There were significant increases in strength and mobility. A study in Japan showed that water exercise, if consistently practiced, also increases bone mineral density and encourages more general daily physical activity. I can corroborate the effectiveness of that type of exercise: my sister-in-law, Ethel Gerstein, who at this writing is eighty-two, in terrific health, takes no medicines, and almost never goes to a doctor, does water aerobics three or four times per week.

One woman I know decided it was time for an exercise program, but she didn't want to spend the money to join a health club, or even to buy dumbbells. So she started lifting kitchen chairs, gallon bottles with water in them, and other heavy household items; I saw her two months after she had put herself on the program and she was feeling and looking happier, peppier, and stronger.

This is no news for most readers, I'm sure; however, a little reminder is always good. And no, there are no exercise pills. We have to do it all ourselves—thirty minutes or so three or four times a week seems to be enough to help keep bones strong. Ideally, you can design an exercise program that combines walking or other exercises that work the legs, weight training, and a flexibility and balance system such as yoga or Tai Chi. On the other hand, excessive physical exercise, such as that pursued by athletes, can interfere with the function of the reproductive system because it may cause excessive leanness; the lack of subcutaneous fat then results in estrogen deficiency and thus in menstrual irregularities and, eventually, possible bone loss.

For inveterate couch potatoes, professional help for anything other than walking would be a good idea. Try the local Y, exercise clubs, books, videos, or a personal trainer until you've set up new habits of healthful movement.

Light and Vitamin D

We do take it totally for granted, but natural light is as much a nutrient as food and water. It is especially important for our bones, as sunlight prods our bodies into producing vitamin D, which is necessary to absorb calcium from the intestines into the blood. According to Micheal F. Holick, the director of the Vitamin D, Skin and Bone Research Laboratory at Boston University Medical Center, about 30 to 40 percent of the people who get hip fractures are vitamin D-deficient. In an interview published in *Nutrition Action*, the health letter of the Center for Science in the Public Interest, he pointed out that regardless of the amount of calcium consumed, this deficiency accelerates bone loss and increases the risk of fractures. To prevent vitamin D deficiency, he recommended to walk with face, hands and arms exposed to the sun, or at least to daylight, two or three times a week, for about half the time it would take for one to get sunburned, or between 10 and 20 minutes, depending on the person, the season, and the distance from the equator. The best time of day for this would be between nine a.m. and four p.m. in the winter, and between eight a.m. and five p.m. in the summer.

Most importantly, Dr. Holick recommended this exposure to the sun be without sunscreen, as sunscreen interferes with the production of vitamin D. An SPF (sun protection factor) of 8 allows only 5 percent of normal production of the vitamin, while with an SPF of 30 there is virtually none produced at all. It is possible to accumulate vitamin D in the tissues during the season with high amounts of sunlight, which can then be used up slowly during the darker months.

Milk is supposedly fortified with vitamin D. However, according to studies published in the *New England Journal of Medicine* in 1991 and 1993, seven out of ten samples of milk contained less than 80 percent of the amount listed on the label, five didn't even have 50 percent, and 14 percent of the skim milk samples had no vitamin D at all. An excellent source is the classic cod liver oil, traditionally used in Northern countries during the winter. And of course, fatty ocean fish such as mackerel and salmon are also traditional sources of vitamin D; two or three servings per week are quite sufficient. Interestingly, Paul Stitt, a biochemist and the author of *Beating the*

Strengthening Bones: The Natural Approach

Best food choices: organically grown or raised, fresh, natural, unrefined foods including whole grains, beans, fresh vegetables, fruits, nuts, seeds, and small amounts of animal foods. Emphasize dark leafy greens, carrots, yams, cruciferous vegetables (broccoli, cabbage, celery).

Include: sea vegetables, soy foods, filtered or spring water.

Calcium-mineral boosters: plant foods, stocks made from bones, healthy fats (see below), small whole fish with bones, canned salmon and sardines with bones, chewing on chicken bones, 15 to 20 minutes of exposure to sunlight three times per week or more.

Healthful fats: modest amounts of extra virgin olive oil, flaxseed oil, unrefined sesame and sunflower oils, traditional coconut and palm oils, organic butter from healthy cows, fish oils. They help the body retain vitamin D, prevent calcium from being excreted in urine. Good-quality saturated fats prevent free radical damage of bones.

Best types of exercise: walking, weight bearing, yoga, Tai Chi—three or more times per week.

Food Giants, reports that the regular consumption of flax seeds increases vitamin D levels as well as the retention of calcium magnesium, and phosphates, which is all good news for the bones. A teaspoon to a tablespoon of flax seeds can be ground in a coffee or spice grinder and added just before serving to porridges, grains, breads, or even drinks.

Now let's see what it takes to reverse osteoporosis. As we shall see, a diagnosis of low bone mass is not the end of the world nor does it inevitably lead to fractures.

7

Can Lost Bone Be Regained?

Dem bones, dem bones gonna rise again . . .
—Old folk spiritual

The answer is yes, but it takes some work. Consider the case of Nina Merer, a New York City stress management consultant and licensed acupressurist, who took some classes with me in the early eighties. She was diagnosed with osteopenia in 1985, at the age of forty; her condition was considered quite advanced, or "almost breakable." After trying prescribed calcium supplements first, but finding herself with too many unpleasant side effects such as intestinal bloating and headaches, she decided to go the "wholistic" route. Her doctor was doubtful, but supportive.

Why did she have such thin bones while she was still premenopausal? Basically, she had a number of risk factors: being quite slim, a Caucasian of Eastern European heritage, with no children, and her mother had osteoporosis. Nina also felt that hard work and play in her twenties and thirties had stressed and depleted her. She had an untreated thyroid condition, many digestive difficulties, food sensitivities, and a feeling of exhaustion. She had also felt an achy, arthritic pain, and a sense "like my bones were falling apart," which finally prompted her to seek professional help.

"It was a depressing diagnosis," she told me in 1997, "but it really served me. I began to think more deeply and decided to take responsibility, prevent further bone loss and to replace what I'd lost." She implemented for herself a five-point program:

1. **Physical.** This included the following:
   - *Exercise.* Having done moderate *weight training* for many

years, Nina now committed herself to a more systematic and intense program. She began *running*, and after becoming a marathoner, she eventually settled into running five miles about four times per week, a moderate distance in the runners' world. She also spent quite a bit of time *stretching*, as she always felt better with it.

• *Acupressure.* Nina used various forms of daily self-help acupressure and got regular sessions from another practitioner, to stimulate her body's energy points. She found it invaluable to both reduce stress and increase energy.

• *Herbs.* Working with a practitioner of Chinese herbal medicine, she started a regime of Chinese herbs to strengthen and tone her system.

• *Food.* Nina's approach was twofold. She eliminated the calcium drainers (caffeine, nightshades, spinach, sugar) and foods she had developed sensitivities to (wheat, oats, barley, rye, corn, dairy, eggs, red meat, vinegar, and fried and fermented foods). She focused on a healthy, whole-foods, balanced diet, using organic foods whenever possible. Her meals consisted of nonglutinous grains (buckwheat, rice, and some millet), fish, organic chicken, some tofu, a little fruit, and, as she put it, "vegetables, vegetables, vegetables." Following her mother Ella's advice, every day she daily had one to three glasses of a mineral-rich blended vegetable drink made with romaine lettuce, carrots, parsley, radish, and celery. (You'll find it in the recipe section under "Green Drink.")

Thirdly, as calcium enrichers, she regularly consumed seaweed, dark greens (collards, kale, mustard greens), and chewed on the bones of chicken and fish, eating the marrow when possible. She also consumed lots of sesame seeds, mainly toasted over her breakfast grain; other seeds she used were chia, sunflower, and fennel. On the whole, she used few spices, no alcohol, and eliminated fruit juices as too sugary. As fats she used borage oil supplements daily (helpful for the bones and to ameliorate arthritis), walnut or canola oil on the salad and sautéed vegetables, soy, and sesame oil also on occasion, and the rare avocado. She'd always had trouble digesting fats, including olive oil, so for a long time she eliminated them from her diet; however, then she started feeling badly in new ways, with more arthritic pains, muscle pain, loss of muscle strength and size, unpleasant menopausal symptoms, and memory loss. When she re-introduced healthy fats into her regime, most of those complaints disappeared.

2. **Hormonal.** Upon entering perimenopause, Nina tried both prescribed birth control pills and hormone replacement therapy (HRT) with the standard drugs, but felt "unacceptably uncomfortable" for six months on them and decided to change course. She read extensively, asked many questions, and with the help of a new and empathetic gynecologist she found the Women's International Pharmacy in Wisconsin, which specializes in soy-based natural hormones in oil capsules. Together they worked on adjusting the doses until they were optimal for her. It was suggested that, instead of taking them by mouth, she open the capsules and put the oil on her skin. Nina felt that this was comfortable and helpful, and a viable solution.

3. **Mental.** Nina found that stress was a major problem in her life. To reduce it, she designed her own serious stress management program which became the foundation of her professional work. In addition to the already mentioned acupressure and exercise, it included affirmations, visualization, meditation, and breathing exercises. Her goal became to simplify and streamline her life, and get her priorities in order. All of these activities helped her become clear and focused, feel better, and, she says, "think straight, which was a major turning point."

4. **Emotional.** Nina found that the physical and mental tools mentioned above were also beneficial emotionally. In addition, she used a system called "reframing" to learn to see obstacles as opportunities for learning. She found that another way to reduce stress is to focus only on solving solvable conflicts, instead of dwelling on things she could do nothing about.

5. **Spiritual.** Attending to her soul's needs, she found that meditation gave her deep satisfaction in new and profound ways. It helped her see the whole picture for better clarity and planning, and find creative solutions to her challenges.

Sounds like a serious, even radical, program, doesn't it? Well, the results astonished her doctor. After twelve years, at fifty-two and already well into menopause, Nina's wrist bone measures over the 100 percent level for her age group, her spine is a bit lower, and her hips are low normal, "fragile but not breakable." She estimates having gained at least ten percent bone density. Now she is classified as "mildly osteopenic." "If I hadn't done something I would have serious osteoporosis," she said. "It took a serious commitment, but I was willing to take a long time to correct a condition that took a lifetime to develop. This was a case of crisis-driven creativity. There are no quick fixes! Once you decide to take charge, it's doable."

We may not all need, want, or be able to spend the time to embark on such an extensive regimen in our own lives, but incorporating even a few of these elements can result in noticeable, positive changes. Here are the seven main physical things to keep in mind for your bone health:

- Avoid sugar, white flour, hydrogenated fats, excess nightshades, fat-free diets, any soft drinks, caffeine, alcohol, smoking
- Avoid excess calcium
- Easy on the milk products—use them only if your ancestors ate them, if you are not lactose intolerant, prone to mucus or infections, or suffering from immune disorders. Limit them to organic butter, plain organic yogurt, unpasteurized cheeses in small amounts on occasion
- Eat daily: Greens and vegetables, some animal food, beans, whole grains, nuts and seeds
- Always cook with stocks
- Walk daily and lift things, or do formal weight training three or more times per week

Finding Our Strength

We can eat lots of greens and take many pills and do all kinds of exercise, but will that be enough to strengthen our bones? If, as I and many others believe, the body and mind-spirit are one, it may not be. Life is hard for most of us; the scant social support we get needs to be boosted thoroughly by our own efforts at believing in ourselves. It's even harder for women who have had no children. First of all, they are told that such a state is already a risk factor for osteoporosis. Secondly, on a subconscious level they have perhaps a need to still look young and attractive in order to attract a mate (whether they have one or not) for procreation.

What we are never told is that there are many ways in which a woman can "give birth" to her creations, be they children, art, books, or businesses. There are many ways in which a woman can use her inborn instinct to nurture, by bringing it to her friends, nephews and nieces, other people's children, staff, coworkers, clients, customers, patients, or pets. By fully accepting our state, whatever it is, by seeing how we have brought ourselves to where we are through our choices *and declaring them good and valid*, we can regain and boost our inner strength and structure. After all, everything is a lesson.

Let's take a look at our personal, emotional, and spiritual support systems, since they will hold up our physical structure—and not the other way around. What follows is my interpretation and synthesis of the work of many masters, principally George Ohsawa's Seven Levels of Judgment and Caroline Myss's philosophical view of the chakras, and its application to our subject.

Our Seven Structures

Everything is connected. As above, so below, and as is the inner, so is the outer. But does the body affect the mind, or the other way around? In body-mind relationships, all questions about causality are chicken-or-egg questions. I think we should consider this a two-way street: the body affects the mind, *and* the mind affects the body. *To make changes, we can start at either end and get results.*

1. **Physical:** *Our Body.* We've been talking about our bones. For a spiritual viewpoint, I look to Rudolf Steiner, the German philosopher and founder of anthroposophy, biodynamic farming, and the Waldorf schools. Thomas Cowan, M.D., a Concord, New Hampshire, physician certified in anthroposophical medicine, wrote that according to Steiner, "One's physical structure is the external manifestation and, in fact, the basis of an orderly thinking process and often an orderly society. Our bones are (or at least were) formed in precise mathematical relationships, which give our subconscious the experience of form, order, and logic."

   Thus, good bones give us a good basis for a coherent and orderly mental and emotional structure, and weak bones will correlate with a lack of inner strength. This lack may have come through early malnutrition, neglect, abuse, or trauma. Recognizing this situation can be of help in motivating us to take care of strengthening our bones through diet and exercise. Then, as the bones get stronger, the rest of us will too.

2. **Tribal:** *Family, Friends, Relationships.* We need this structure for our sense of connection and belonging within a recognizable group of

people, who can give us support and receive ours in turn. If we have no mate or immediate family around, we need to create a structure of friends and coworkers that give us that essential sense of tribal unity, without which loneliness can be truly unbearable.

3. **Emotional:** *Sense of Self.* Knowing "who we are" in terms of that sense of "I am who I am" is necessary as an inner structure to withstand the inevitable emotional blows that life sends our way. Any time we feel the need to ask "who am I?" we can assume that this sense is wobbly.

4. **Intellectual:** *Work, Hobbies, Study.* Being gainfully employed, or occupied in regular and satisfying activities is what we need to give structure to our days as well as our intellectual and creative energies. This is not only about making a living, it's about being involved in something that helps us grow, as well as studying subjects that interest us. Having nothing to do is demoralizing and lowers our self-esteem, regardless of the thickness of our wallet.

5. **Social:** *Community, Ecology.* We need to feel and understand that we are part of a larger community, part of this world, and that our actions impact our environment. Chaos theory, one of the more interesting models in theoretical physics, states that everything is connected, and small disturbances in one area of the whole can create large and unexpected outcomes elsewhere: in other words, the beating of a butterfly's wings in Tokyo can eventually loosen a storm upon New York. We are part of the larger structure of our world, and need to be conscious of that to find a larger meaning in our lives, to know that we matter.

6. **Philosophical:** *A View of Life.* This to me is an essential component of our total structure, an understanding or simply a model of how the world works, that will help us figure things out, make decisions, predict what is going to happen if we follow one course over another. Religions will often provide a view of life for a large majority of people. ("If you do this, then thus and such will happen," e.g., if you misbehave, don't follow the rules, you will be punished.) Many of us also put together our own worldview. I find that building a cohesive one is one of the more fun activities of my life.

7. **Spiritual:** *A Connection with the Divine or the Transcendental.* A feeling of awe tells us when we reach that connection. For our spiritual structure, we need to know that there is something unfathomable about the world we live in, that there is always a mystery and an exquisite order far beyond our ken, and that we are still a part of it.

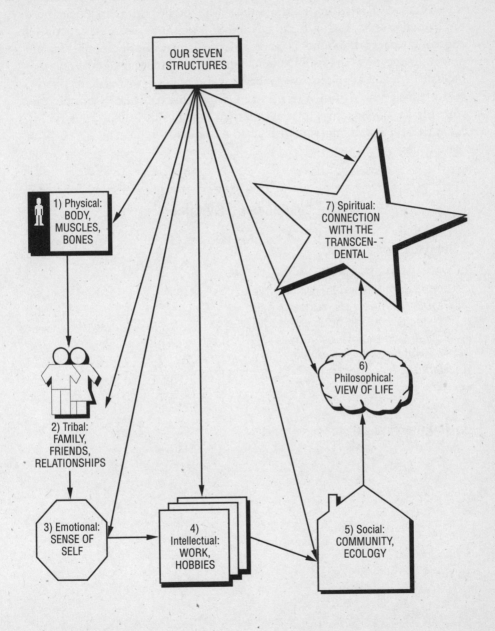

Do you recognize an emptiness, a lack in any of the above structures in your life? If you often worry about your bones, look into these subjects as well. Number 1 is addressed throughout this book. Numbers 2, 3, and 4 can be addressed through therapy. Number 5 requires community activism and volunteer work. Numbers 6 and 7 need introspection, meditation, and prayer. In addition, the Five Element Theory in Chinese medicine says that excess worry is, like excess sweets, bad for the bones—therefore, it is helpful to banish worry from your life as much as possible. Just as you increase your intake of vegetables to strengthen your bones as well as your health, consider also increasing your overall inner stability by attending to all of these issues.

Can Lost Bone Be Regained?

Bones are part of our whole being. To keep them strong, we must attend to all our aspects:

Physical: Body and bones
Tribal: Family, friends, relationships
Emotional: Feelings, sense of self
Intellectual: Work, hobbies, study
Social: Community, ecology
Philosophical: A view of life
Spiritual: A connection with the transcendental or divine

And now, let's cook.

8

Recipes for Strong Bones

We all begin as a bundle of bones lost somewhere in a desert, a dismantled skeleton that lies under the sand. It is our work to recover the parts.

—Clairissa Pinkola Estes,
Women Who Run with the Wolves

Traditional cuisines generally are rich in all essential nutrients, from both animal and vegetable sources. However, every culture has very specific considerations regarding which foods are edible and which are not. The most stringent restrictions are those relating to animal products; those culturally rejected are often considered "unclean." For example, in Western culture we eat cow, chicken, turkey, lamb, fish, and to a lesser degree rabbit, quail, deer, and wild game. We do not eat dog, elephant, monkey, or insects, because we consider them distasteful, even though these are consumed in many other countries. Certain religions are very specific regarding what is edible: according to the Jewish kosher laws, pork and shellfish are unclean, and the Muslim custom also eschews pork. These prohibitions have nothing to do with nutrition (insects, for example, are an excellent source of minerals!) but are simply cultural conditioning. In our contemporary society, even animal foods that were common up to forty or fifty years ago are now often considered unpleasant: tongue, heart, kidneys, tripe, bone marrow. Many traditional recipes are very high in minerals: calf's foot jelly, oxtail stew, bird's nest soup, pig's head, fried ants. Nevertheless, we will not see these in popular restaurants or modern cookbooks, due to changing tastes and political sensibilities.

The narrowing of the national diet in the United States has a lot to do with advertising and marketing. In a country that has such an abundant quantity of food, it's remarkable that people restrict themselves to mostly hamburgers, hot dogs, pasta, pizza, chicken, and ice cream. And let's not forget snack foods. I once saw a statistic that pointed out that on any given day, 26 percent of the population doesn't eat a single vegetable. I believe it, too. It's because we never see any ads for really good, fresh vegetable dishes, only for the frozen or canned variety, which are never as good as fresh. No famous sports figures or movie stars promote them. This relentless advertising has changed the nature of what we eat so that most people are content with packaged, colored, flavored, and otherwise doctored-up foods, even while their bodies are starved for natural nutrients. The habit of continuous snacking just indicates how hungry people are, and the snacking itself does not satisfy that hunger but worsens it. Such a situation is all the better for the food giants and all the worse for our bodies.

Another reason why our food is less nutritious is commercial farming and animal husbandry. Traditional organic farming methods using compost and manure return a rich mix of nutrients to the soil. Twentieth-century commercial petroleum-based or mineral fertilizers only add a few specific minerals. As a result, tests are now finding that organically grown vegetables are 50 to 150 percent higher in nutrients than commercial produce. Animals that are raised with synthetic foods, antibiotics, and hormones often are not as healthy as animals that roam in the wild eating their natural foods; chemical residues may remain in their tissues that are then consumed by the public. Obviously, most people don't fall over dead when they eat these commercial foods, so there is a lot of questioning whether these chemical additives really pose a hazard. I say, in the long run, they probably do—and that is hard to prove with the scientific method because we'd have to study a very large group of people (many thousands) over one or two generations, and I venture it would be almost impossible to find such a large group that only eats organically grown food with no deviations for twenty-five years. Just to be safe, whenever we have the choice I believe it's best to go for the organically grown or raised, free-range, chemical-free, natural foods. At the very least, they taste better.

I realize that most people are very busy, and have "no time" to devote to cooking for themselves. That may be fine while one is reasonably healthy, but will we stay well on such a diet of lifeless foods? I truly have my doubts. The compromise that I suggest is to cook planning to have plenty of leftovers, maybe two or three times per week, and keeping the foods in the fridge, not the freezer, until they're used up. Even if we don't eat three home-cooked meals each day, at least let's eat one or two. While it's impossible to get whole grains in a coffee shop, let's have some oatmeal or kasha or brown rice or whole-grain bread at home. The time we invest in insuring we have healthful food available is time invested in our own and our family's health. Healthy people cost less money than sick people! Therefore, cooking healthful food is a good investment, in terms of both time and money.

The recipes that follow were created to maximize the intake of minerals, essential fatty acids, fiber, complex carbohydrates, and good-quality protein. They are *not* skewed for maximum calcium only, but for well-rounded nutrition. There are both vegetarian and animal protein–based choices. Most of the recipes will come with some suggestion of how or with what to serve them. All grain and bean recipes, as well as soups, keep really well in the refrigerator for four to five days. Animal food recipes are best eaten within two days.

Nutrition Information

Most of the nutrition information for these recipes was obtained through a computer program, the *FoodProcessor for Windows*, version 7. However, there were a number of dishes that I had analyzed privately. To help you see their full nutritional value, in appendix A you will find, for each recipe, a complete listing and bar graph of all the essential nutrients as compared to the needs of a fifty-five-year-old, 5′4″, 150-lb. woman. You may be far on either side of this "average," you may not even be a woman, but the graph is a dramatic visual depiction that will give you a basic idea of the percentages as well as the actual amounts of each nutrient. You will also find sample breakfast, lunch, and dinner menus, as well as two "whole day" analyses.

Please note that while the program considers 800 milligrams of calcium the optimum amount, according to figures mentioned earlier, in this type of nutritious diet 450 to 500 mg can be considered sufficient. As you will see, this is easily attainable. If in your personal case you need a higher amount of calcium, and if you have no objection to milk products, you can add a slice or two of natural cheese to boost your intake of that mineral. Or you can work with a nutritionist or other knowledgeable health professional and come up with a supplementation program individually tailored to your needs. I do not recommend that you take any supplements shotgun or "just in case," or simply from a book, as I believe that they could confuse your body if you don't happen to need them.

Ingredients

I use the following parameters to guide me in the choice of ingredients:

- The best choice is always organically grown grains, beans, vegetables, fruits.
- Whenever possible, choose fresh wild fish and free-range or organically raised fowl, eggs, and meats.
- The best-quality fats are extra virgin olive oil, unrefined sesame oil, and organic unsalted butter—all to be used in sufficient quantity to make the food satisfying.

However, remember also that our choices are not always perfect. If the option is between commercially raised foods and nothing, please eat what is available, and with gratitude!

There are a few ingredients in these recipes that need some explanation.

- *Water.* Clean filtered, artesian, or spring water is always preferable to chlorinated and fluoridated city water. There are many types of water filters on the market, certainly one for every budget. There are filters in a jar that you can keep in the refrigerator, others that are hooked up to the faucet, to the water supply under the sink, or even to the water supply of the whole house. I personally prefer to purchase natural spring water in five-gallon bottles, and use that for all cooking and drinking.
- *Sea vegetables or seaweeds.* These are plants that grow in the sea, and coastal cultures such as the Irish and the Japanese have long used them in their cuisines. They are very high in calcium and other minerals, and so an excellent addition to a healthful cuisine. They also contain iodine, which is necessary for the thyroid in small amounts. I often find that people who have low thyroid function love sea vegetables! Because they are so rich, they're best used in small amounts. The main varieties are kombu, wakame, hiziki, arame, kanten (or agar, used for thickening like gelatin), and dulse.
- *Umeboshi vinegar.* This is a Japanese product that I find extremely useful for seasoning soups, stews, dressings, dips, and spreads. It is a by-product of the manufacture of *umeboshi plums*, which are plums pickled in brine for two years or so. Umeboshi vinegar is both salty and sour, and imparts a light and delightful touch to otherwise dense or heavy foods.

- *Kuzu.* A starch extracted from the root of the kudzu plant, originally from Japan, this white chunky powder is similar in action to cornstarch or arrowroot. However, it has a small amount of calcium, a neutral taste making it ideal to thicken almost anything, and a nice smooth texture when properly prepared. It is also very soothing to the stomach.

All these ingredients can be found in health food markets or supermarkets with Asian or natural food sections.

Staples to Keep on Hand in Your Kitchen

Whole grains: oatmeal, brown rice, whole wheat flour, kasha, millet, barley
Beans: lentils, navy beans, pinto beans, chickpeas, red lentils
Produce: onions, garlic, carrots, celery, parsley
Seasonings and cooking aids: extra virgin olive oil, unrefined sesame oil, flaxseed oil, natural soy sauce, balsamic or brown rice vinegar, umeboshi vinegar, sea salt
Herbs: oregano, basil, thyme, tarragon, rosemary, sage
Spices: cinnamon, nutmeg, cloves, turmeric, cumin (ground and seeds), ginger powder, cardamom pods, coriander (ground and seeds)
Nuts and seeds: almonds, sunflower seeds, sesame seeds, walnuts (store nuts in the freezer to keep them fresh)
Snacks: rye crackers, whole wheat crackers, dates, raisins
Stocks: vegetable, chicken, fish

Stocks

Stocks are one of the best ways to get minerals into your system. They enrich the nutrient value of every dish and deepen the flavor. Fine chefs spend much time and attention on their stocks. "My stocks are like gold to me," says Lauren Groveman, a cooking teacher in Westchester, New York, and author of *Lauren Groveman's Kitchen.*

They can be made with scraps and leftover vegetables and bones from fish, fowl, or meat. Basic vegetables include onions, carrots, celery, leek and scallion tops, turnips, parsley stems; they can be a little old, wilted, or ugly, as long as they're not moldy. Avoid the cruciferous vegetables, such as broccoli, cabbage, cauliflower, and kale; they are too sulfuric and give an unpleasantly strong odor when cooked for a long time. Avoid also the top half inch of carrots, where the carrot meets the leaf stem; that part is very bitter and can give a terribly harsh flavor to the stock that cannot be disguised.

Good Stock Vegetables *(mild-tasting)*

carrots	scallion tops
onions	garlic cloves
onion skins (will make stock brown)	shallots
celery	mushrooms and stems
celery tops (if organic)	zucchini
parsley stems	string bean tips
turnips	
leek tops	

Vegetables to Avoid for Stock
(strong-tasting, bitter, or with deep color)

broccoli	cabbage leaves	potato skins
broccoli leaves	Brussels sprouts	eggplant
cauliflower	kohlrabi	parsley leaves
cauliflower leaves	mustard greens	beets and greens
kale	yams	green or red peppers
collards	sweet potatoes	
cabbage	potatoes	

When making stock with bones, always add a tablespoon of vinegar or a half cup of wine for every two quarts of water to leach the calcium and other minerals out of the bones, and make them available in the stock. (This need not be done with vegetables.) To increase the mineral content without adding odd flavors, you can add one tablespoon agar seaweed (available in health food stores) to each quart of cold stock before using (see appendix A for nutrient analysis). The stocks I had analyzed ranged between 5 and 15 mg of calcium and 3 to 9 mg of magnesium per 100 grams.

On the whole, stocks are not a significant source of fats and contain no protein. Once they're made, they can be frozen in quart or pint plastic containers, or in ice cube trays. The stock ice cubes can be placed in zippered plastic bags or other containers, to be retrieved as needed.

Make a minimum of two quarts of stock each time; more is even better. Frozen stock keeps well for about three months. In the refrigerator, vegetable or chicken stock can be kept for about a week, but it needs to be brought to a boil every three days. Any time a stock is thawed from frozen, it also needs to be brought to a rolling boil to eliminate any bacteria that might have appeared, and to bring it to life, in a way, after such a long hibernation.

The following stocks were made exactly according to the recipes. However, in making stock do not be bound by strict recipes, but follow the basic concept. Essentially, you start with a few vegetables and scraps, a bouquet garni, or collection of spices and herbs, and, depending on the stock, some bones and vinegar or wine. Add enough water to cover by three inches, and simmer with the cover ajar for an hour or more. Particularly with bone-based stocks, the longer you cook them the richer they get. You can leave the cover off for the last half hour so as to concentrate the stock; that way you will have less to store in the freezer. *Never salt a stock;* as stocks are ingredients in other recipes, it's best that the salting be done in the final cooking.

If you give yourself four hours or so, you can make two or three quarts each of two different types of stock—say, vegetable and chicken—which can last you between a week and a month, depending on how often you cook and for how many people. I promise you that making stocks is worth the investment of your time and effort, both in nutrition and in flavor. Your health, and your bones, will be grateful.

If it is impossible for you to make homemade stocks, the only acceptable substitute in my opinion is fresh, concentrated, or frozen stocks made with natural ingredients by a chef in a restaurant or local food store. For example, a food store I frequent in Manhattan, Citarella, has excellent freshly made fish, chicken, and beef stocks, and even demi-glace, a classic French thick and gelatinous concentrated veal stock, used in sauces. I would stay away from dried and cubed bouillons, which are mostly salt, MSG, and flavorings, and do not in any way contribute minerals to your meal except sodium.

Simple Vegetable Stock

This is an easy stock to have on hand. Sautéing the vegetables gives it a deeper and fuller flavor, but if you're in a rush you can skip that step.

1	medium onion, cut up (about 1 cup)
2	medium carrots, scrubbed and cut into chunks (about 1 cup)
2	celery ribs, with leaves if organic, sliced into chunks
1	leek
1	tablespoon extra virgin olive oil
1	piece kombu seaweed (about 3 inches)
3	garlic cloves, peeled, sliced
1/2	cup parsley stems
2	bay leaves
1/2	teaspoon dried thyme
1	teaspoon mixed white and black peppercorns
6	cups cold water

1. Wash and prep the vegetables. Slice the leek in half lengthwise, then chop crosswise into 1/4-inch slices. Use as much of the greens as possible; discard the really tough and ugly leaves. Drop the chopped leeks into a bowl of cold water and swish around until they feel clean. Allow to settle for a moment, then fish out the leeks with your hands and put them in another bowl, leaving behind the sand and grit.
2. In a 4-quart stockpot, heat the oil, then add the onion, carrots, celery, and leek. Sauté over medium heat until they soften and become aromatic; do not brown. Add the kombu, garlic, seasonings, and water. Bring to a simmer, and cook over low heat for about 1 hour, with the cover ajar.
3. Strain the stock through a fine strainer, pressing on the vegetables with a ladle or wooden spoon to extract all the liquid. Don't press so much as to push the vegetables themselves through the strainer. Cool and store.

Makes about 1 quart

Rich Vegetable Stock

This stock will have a little oil in it, both from the walnuts and from the olive oil, which are rich in essential fatty acids. Don't try to remove it.

1   large onion, cut up (about 1 cup)
2   carrots, cut into chunks (about 1 cup)
2   celery stalks, cut into 1/2-inch pieces (1 cup)
1   medium leek (1/2 cup), cleaned and sliced (see page 102)
1   turnip, cut into medium dice (1/2 cup)
1/4 cup walnuts
10   mushrooms with stems (old ones are fine), sliced
11/2 tablespoons extra virgin olive oil
1   piece kombu seaweed (about 5 inches)
1/4 cup white beans, soaked 8 hours, drained
4   quarts cold water

Bouquet garni

1/4 cup parsley stems (no leaves)
1   bay leaf
1   teaspoon sage
1   teaspoon thyme
1/2 teaspoon peppercorns

1. Preheat the oven to 450 degrees F.
2. Wash and chop the vegetables.
3. Place the onion, carrots, celery, leek, turnip, mushrooms, and walnuts in an 11 × 15-inch baking pan and drizzle with the oil. Toss well, until every piece is coated with the oil. Place in the preheated oven and roast for about 20 minutes, or until lightly browned. Turn the vegetables over with a spatula every 5 to 6 minutes, so they cook evenly. (This step may be omitted for a light-colored stock.)
4. Place the roasted vegetables, kombu, drained beans, and water into a 6- or 8-quart stockpot. Add a little water to the baking pan to deglaze it and pick up the brown bits and juices; scrape the bottom with a metal spatula if needed. Pour into the stockpot. Place the bouquet garni ingredients on a 6 × 6-inch piece of cheesecloth and tie into a bundle; add to the pot.
5. Bring to a boil, then simmer for 11/2 hours with the cover ajar. Remove any foam or scum that comes to the surface during the cooking. Make

sure it simmers very slowly; don't keep at a rolling boil. Leave the cover off for the last $1/2$ hour so as to concentrate the stock.

6. Remove and discard the bouquet garni. Strain the stock through a fine strainer, pressing the solids with the back of a ladle or wooden spoon to extract all the liquids. Cool and store.

Makes about 2 quarts

Simple Chicken Stock I

1   medium onion, peeled, cut in half
1   small carrot, 1/2 inch removed from the top, cut into large
     chunks
4   garlic cloves, peeled and smashed
1   celery stalk or 3 to 4 celery tops (organic only)
     Carcass and bones of 1 organic or free-range chicken (about
     1 pound), with or without skin
3   quarts cold water
2   tablespoons brown rice or apple cider vinegar
1   large bay leaf
1   teaspoon dried basil
1/4   teaspoon black peppercorns

1. Wash and chop the vegetables.
2. Place all the ingredients in a 6- to 8-quart stockpot over low heat, and allow to come barely to a simmer. Cook with the cover ajar for about 2 hours; do not boil. Remove the cover, then cook for 1 hour more. Strain without pushing the solids to get a very clear, unclouded stock. Chill and remove the congealed fat before freezing. Freeze in plastic containers or ice cube trays, or store in the refrigerator and use within 3 days.

Makes about 2 quarts

Gourmet Chicken Stock II

1   large onion, coarsely chopped (about 1 cup)
2   small carrots, cut into chunks (about 1 cup)
2   celery ribs, cut into 1/2-inch slices (about 1 cup)
1   small leek, cleaned and thinly sliced (see page 102)
1   turnip, cut into medium dice (about 1/2 cup)
2   ounces button mushrooms, sliced (about 1/2 cup)
2   tablespoons apple cider or balsamic vinegar
    Bouquet garni (see page 103)
2   bay leaves
1/2 teaspoon dry rosemary
1   teaspoon thyme
3   cardamom pods
1   teaspoon peppercorns
    Backbones, neck, and wingtips of one free-range or organic
       chicken, washed, with skin
    Carcass and bones from one cooked free-range or organic
       chicken
4   quarts cold water, or enough to cover by 3 inches

1. Wash and chop the vegetables.
2. Place all the ingredients in a 6- or 8-quart stockpot over low heat, and allow to come barely to a simmer. Cook with the cover ajar for about 2 hours; do not boil. Remove the cover, then cook for 2 to 3 hours more. Strain without pushing the solids to get a clear, unclouded stock. Chill and remove the congealed fat before freezing. Freeze in plastic containers or ice cube trays, or store in the refrigerator and use within 3 days.

Makes about 2 quarts

Fish Stock

Purchase the whole fish and have it filleted at the store. Ask them to place the bones in one bag, the fillets in another. Use the bones for the stock, the fillets broiled for lunch or dinner, or in the soup.

       Heads, bones, and tails of two 10- to 12-inch mild fish
          (snapper, bass, sole)
       Greens of 1 leek, chopped
       Greens of 5 scallions, chopped
1   carrot, sliced (about 1 cup)
1   large onion, coarsely chopped (about 1 cup)
1   tablespoon apple cider or balsamic vinegar, or 1/2 cup white
      wine
       Bouquet garni (see page 103)
1/4 cup parsley stems (do not use leaves, they make the stock
      green)
1   bay leaf
1   teaspoon dry oregano
1   teaspoon dry thyme
1/2 teaspoon peppercorns
4   quarts cold water

1. Wash the bones in several changes of water, until the water is no longer cloudy. Soak them in the last change of water until you finish prepping the vegetables.
2. Wash and chop the vegetables.
3. Place the fish bones, vegetables, vinegar, bouquet garni, and water in a 6- to 8-quart stockpot. Bring to a boil, lower the heat, and simmer for 45 to 50 minutes with the cover ajar. Remove the cover for the last 15 minutes to concentrate the stock.
4. Strain, pushing the solids into the strainer so as to extract all the nutrient-rich liquid. Cool. Freeze in plastic containers or ice cube trays, or store in the refrigerator and use within 3 days.

Makes about 2 1/2 quarts

Shrimp Stock

Clean and devein the shrimp, and use them in bisques or stir-fries. Use the shells for the stock.

       Shells and tails from 2 pounds medium shrimp
1   large onion, chopped (about 1 cup)
2   celery ribs, sliced (about 1 cup)
1   tablespoon peppercorns
1/8 teaspoon dried tarragon
1   bay leaf
2^1/2 cups Fish Stock (see page 107)
6^1/2 cups cold water
1/2 cup white wine, or 1 tablespoon apple cider vinegar

1. Wash the shells. Wash and prep the vegetables.
2. Place all the ingredients in a 3-quart stockpot. Bring to a boil, lower the heat, and simmer for 1^1/2 hours with the cover ajar.
3. Strain, pushing the solids into the strainer with the back of a ladle to extract all the nutrient-rich stock. Use immediately, or store in the freezer.

Makes about 2 quarts

Kombu Stock

2^1/2 cups water
1   stick dried kombu seaweed
1   tablespoon bonita fish flakes (obtainable in Japanese or
     natural food stores)

1. In a 1- or 2-quart saucepan, bring the water to a boil and add kombu. Simmer five minutes, covered.
2. Add the bonita flakes, turn off the heat, and let the flakes sink to the bottom of the pot. Let sit a minute, then strain. Use immediately. (The kombu and flakes can be re-used one time by simmering them in 2 cups water for ten minutes.)

Beef Stock

The marrow of bones is extremely high in calcium, together with fat, iron, and zinc. In fact, marrow has three times more calcium than milk, ounce for ounce. If you like, you can scrape it out of the bones after the stock is cooked, and spread it on toast with a little salt and pepper. It used to be a common food fifty or so years ago.

2   pounds beef marrow bones (available at the grocery store, or
    ask your butcher)
4   quarts water
1   large carrot, cut up
1   medium onion, cut into quarters
2   celery stalks, cut up
3   garlic cloves, peeled
2   tablespoons olive oil
1/2   cup parsley stems
1   cup red or white wine, or 2 tablespoons wine vinegar

1. Place the bones in a 6- to 8-quart stockpot with the water, bring to a boil, and simmer for 10 minutes. Skim off as much of the scum as possible. Meanwhile, wash and chop the vegetables.
2. Add the vegetables, oil, parsley, and wine to the pot, and simmer on *very low* heat for 2 to 3 hours, with the cover ajar. Skim occasionally.
3. Strain without pushing on the solids. Chill and remove the congealed fat. Freeze or store in the refrigerator and use within 3 days.

Makes about 2^1/$_2$ quarts

Soups

I love soups. When you're really hungry, there is nothing like a flavorful hot soup to soothe a growling stomach. Chilled soups in the summer are cooling and refreshing, hot soups in the winter are an excellent defense against the cold. Soups can be a really easy way to get vegetables into people. Those that are stock based and contain no starchy ingredients like flour, grains, or beans, are excellent alkalizers and counteract the acidifying effects of breads and pastas. Those that contain starches and proteins such as beans, fish, chicken, or meat can be great one-pot meals when accompanied by a salad. In addition, they're a great catchall for odds and ends in the refrigerator: sometimes the best soups are those made with various leftovers and some good stock—and they generally can't be duplicated!

Once you understand the basics of soup making, you'll find endless variations on your favorites. Don't hesitate to experiment!

Cilantro–Egg Drop Soup

Here is a quick, simple, and delicious soup. Serve for a light spring lunch with whole-grain rye bread or crackers, Sardine Spread (page 162), and Asparagus with Slivered Almonds (page 131). For a variation, add 1/2 cup of any leftover cooked vegetable (chopped) or grain.

2 1/2   cups chicken stock
1/4   teaspoon sea salt
1   organic egg, well beaten
2   tablespoons chopped fresh cilantro (coriander leaves or Chinese parsley)
   freshly ground pepper to taste

1. Place the stock and salt in a 2- or 3-quart saucepan and bring to a boil.
2. Beat the egg with a fork in a small bowl. Slowly add to the boiling stock, reduce the heat, and stir continuously with the fork until the egg is cooked firm and stands out from the stock, about 1 minute. Serve immediately, with a tablespoon of cilantro on each serving and freshly ground pepper.

Makes 2 servings

Pinto Bean Soup with Dill

1   tablespoon extra virgin olive oil
1   medium onion, finely diced (about 2 cups)
1   small carrot, diced (about 1 cup)
2   celery ribs, finely diced (about 1 cup)
1   teaspoon ground cumin
1   teaspoon turmeric
4   cups vegetable, chicken, or beef stock or water
1   cup dried pinto beans, soaked 8 hours in 4 cups water, drained
1   tablespoon agar flakes
1   teaspoon sea salt
4   teaspoons fresh chopped dill or cilantro

1. Heat the oil in a 4-quart soup pot, and add the onion, carrot, and celery, sautéing for about 1 minute each before adding the next vegetable. Add the cumin and turmeric, mix well, and sauté another 30 to 40 seconds.
2. Add the stock, beans, and agar, bring to a boil, and simmer, covered, for about 1 hour. Stir every 15 minutes or so. When the beans are soft, add the salt and continue cooking for another 15 minutes.
3. Serve hot, with a teaspoon of fresh dill for garnish.

Makes about 4 servings

Gumbo

This is a meat-free variation on the popular Southern thick soup. If you wish, you can add cooked fish, seafood, or chicken to the end product, simmering an extra 5 minutes, to approximate the original. It's a great dish over rice or other grains, served with a salad or garlic greens.

- 2   leeks
- 1   cup onion, coarsely diced
- 1   small carrot, cut into chunks
- 1   celery stalk, coarsely diced
- 2   garlic cloves, coarsely chopped
- 2   cups vegetable, fish, or chicken stock
- 1   bay leaf
- 1/4   cup dried porcini mushrooms (optional)
- 3   tablespoons clarified butter (see page 114)
- 1/2   teaspoon cumin seeds
- 4   tablespoons buckwheat or whole wheat pastry flour (see Note)
- 1   cup boiling water
- 1   teaspoon sea salt, or to taste
  freshly ground pepper

1. Cut the roots off the leeks and discard. Cut the leeks lengthwise, then across into 1/4-inch slices, starting at the bottom; discard the tough greens as you progress upward, keeping those green parts that are pliable and tender. (Keep the discarded greens for stock.) Put all the leek slices in a large bowl of cold water; stir around with your hand to loosen up the grit and dirt. Scoop the floating leeks out and place in a colander or bowl, leaving the grit in the bottom of the bowl. Rinse out the bowl, add cold water again, and repeat the process with the leeks until they are well cleaned (one or two more times).

2. Place the leeks, onion, carrot, celery, garlic, stock, and bay leaf in a 4-quart soup pot. Break the dried mushrooms, if using, into small pieces and add to the stock. Simmer, half covered, for about 15 minutes.

3. Heat the clarified butter in another saucepan, add the cumin seeds, and stir for a minute or two until fragrant. Add the buckwheat or pastry flour, and stir for 3 to 4 minutes. Whisk in the boiling water and stir until thick and all lumps have disappeared. Simmer a minute, then scrape into the soup pot. Stir well.

4. Add salt and simmer the soup, with the cover on, for 10 to 15 minutes, stirring occasionally. Adjust the seasonings. Serve hot with freshly ground pepper.

Makes 3 to 4 servings

Note: Buckwheat flour gives the soup a dark brown color and deeper flavor; whole wheat pastry flour is lighter.

Clarified Butter (Ghee)

A revered food in India and traditionally used in French cuisine as a standard cooking medium, clarified butter has several advantages. First, it does not go rancid easily and can be kept unrefrigerated in a dark and airtight container for about 3 months. Because the milk solids have been removed, it can be heated to a higher temperature than butter without smoking. In addition, and for the same reason, people allergic to milk protein can generally consume clarified butter.

1   **pound organic unsalted butter**

1. In a small 1-quart saucepan, heat the butter gently over low heat until melted. Allow it to foam for a while as it simmers for about 10 minutes. Spoon off the foam, which contains some of the milk solids. Turn off the heat, and let sit for 3 minutes.
2. Line a fine strainer with two layers of wet cheesecloth and place over a bowl or container (I like to keep ghee in a stone pot with a tight-fitting lid). Carefully strain the clear butterfat through the strainer, leaving behind the bottom residue to discard. Cover the container, and open only briefly to access the contents. The container for the clarified butter should be opaque; if all you have is glass, surround it with aluminum foil to keep out the light, which could cause rancidity. Do not use plastic containers.

Cucumber-Avocado Soup

This is a great cold soup for a summer lunch, a good source of omega-3 and omega-6 fatty acids. Accompany it with some steamed shrimp and corn on the cob. If you make extra, have the leftover soup for a refreshing breakfast or snack on a hot day.

1   garlic clove, peeled
1   large organic cucumber, peeled and seeded, then sliced
        (about $1/2$ pound)
1   teaspoon lemon juice or umeboshi vinegar
2   tablespoons flaxseed, ground fine in a coffee grinder
$3/4$ cup chicken or vegetable stock, or cold water
$1/2$ small Haas (black-skinned) avocado
$1/2$ teaspoon chopped fresh mint leaves

1. Remove the measuring cap from the cover of a blender; place the cover on the blender. Start the machine, and drop in the garlic clove. When it is minced fully, add the cucumber slices one by one. When the mixture gets thick, add the lemon juice or umeboshi vinegar, flaxseed, and stock or water.
2. Add the avocado. Puree until smooth. Thin with a tablespoon of stock or water if too thick. Serve garnished with chopped mint.

Makes 2 servings

Cabbage and Celery Soup

Easy, warming, nutritious, and economical, this is the kind of soup I can live on. Serve it with Polenta with black olives (page 151) and the Chickpea Tabbouleh (page 124) for a nice light meal.

1/2   tablespoon extra virgin olive oil
1   medium onion, chopped (about 1 cup)
2   cups shredded cabbage (about 1/4 large head)
1   teaspoon ground cumin
1   teaspoon sea salt
1   carrot, cut into matchsticks (about 1/2 cup)
3   celery stalks (about 1 cup)
6   cups stock
     freshly ground pepper

1. In a 4-quart saucepan, heat the oil, add the onion, and sauté for 1 to 2 minutes, or until transparent. Add the cabbage, cumin, and salt, and stir until wilted, 2 to 3 minutes. Then add the carrot and celery, and sauté everything for another 5 minutes.
2. Add the stock and simmer, covered, for 35 to 40 minutes. Add a little more stock if needed, adjust the seasoning, and serve hot, with a sprinkle of freshly ground pepper.

Makes 6 servings

Miso Soup with Wild Mushrooms and Garlic

If you like wild mushrooms, you'll love this simple, easy soup. Try it in a meal with Poached Red Snapper Fillets with Parsley Sauce (page 159), plain brown rice (page 146), Puree of Yams (page 142), and Basic Garlic Greens (page 132).

- 1 cup dried mushrooms (any combination of shiitake, porcini, chanterelles, maitake)
- 2 cups fish stock or kombu stock or water
- 4 garlic cloves, minced
- 1/4 cup mellow barley or rice miso
- 1 scallion, whites and greens, sliced thinly on the diagonal

1. Soak the mushrooms in the stock or water for 45 minutes to 1 hour. Drain, reserving the liquid. Cut the stems off the shiitake (reserve the stems for stock). Slice all mushrooms into thin strips.
2. Measure the reserved liquid and add enough water to make 3 cups. Place the liquid in a 4-quart soup pot, then add the mushrooms and garlic. Simmer over medium-low heat for about 30 minutes.
3. Place the miso in a small bowl. Add 1/4 cup of liquid from the soup pot, and blend the miso until creamy. Add to the soup, and simmer another 2 minutes. Serve hot, garnished with 1/2 teaspoon scallion slices.

Makes about 4 servings

Chicken Soup

Here's an easy version of the universal comfort food, which can also provide richly alkalizing minerals.

4	cups chicken stock
2	thighs of a free-range or organic chicken, skinless
2	carrots, peeled and cut into 1-inch dice
1/2	teaspoon sea salt, or to taste
	freshly ground pepper
2	teaspoons chopped fresh parsley
2	teaspoons fresh chives, snipped into 1/4-inch pieces

1. Place the stock, chicken thighs, and carrots in a 2- or 3-quart saucepan. Add the salt and simmer covered, for 25 to 30 minutes.
2. Remove the chicken thighs, pick the meat off the bones, pull or cut it into small pieces, and return it to the soup pot; freeze the bones for stock.
3. Taste, and adjust the seasoning. Serve with some freshly ground pepper and a garnish of parsley and chives in each bowl.

Makes about 4 servings

Spanish Fish Soup

This delicious and easy soup is excellent for company. Serve over brown rice or kasha, or with some good crusty whole-grain bread, a side of Greek olives, and a salad.

2	tablespoons extra virgin olive oil
1	medium onion, chopped
3	garlic cloves, chopped
1/4	teaspoon dried tarragon
3	cups fish stock
	large pinch saffron, crumbled
1	teaspoon salt
4	calamari (squid), cleaned and sliced into rings
1/2	pound small scallops
8	clams
1	pound fresh scrod (or other thick whitefish)
2	teaspoons chopped fresh parsley
	freshly ground black pepper

1. In a large soup pot, heat the oil, add the onion, garlic, and tarragon, and sauté for 2 to 3 minutes, or until fragrant but not browned.
2. Add the stock, saffron, and salt, and simmer, covered, for 20 to 25 minutes. (You can make ahead up to this point.)
3. About 15 minutes before serving, make sure the stock is simmering. Add the calamari and simmer covered, for 3 minutes. Then add the scallops, clams, and scrod, and simmer another 5 to 6 minutes, until the clams are all open (discard clams that do not open after this time).
4. Ladle into bowls over rice or kasha, and garnish each serving with 1/4 teaspoon parsley and some freshly ground pepper.

Makes about 4 servings

Hearty Shrimp Bisque

 3   tablespoons extra virgin olive oil
1/2   cup onion, minced
1/4   cup carrot, finely diced
1/4   cup celery, finely diced
 4   tablespoons whole wheat flour
1/2   cup white wine or water
3 1/2 cups shrimp stock
 1   teaspoon sea salt, or to taste
      pinch saffron
1/2   teaspoon dried thyme
 1   bay leaf
24   fresh shrimp, peeled
 2   teaspoons fresh chives, snipped into 1/2-inch pieces
      freshly ground black pepper to taste

1. In a 4-quart soup pot, heat the oil, add the onion, carrot, and celery, and stir over medium heat. Cover and cook over low heat for 6 to 8 minutes, or until soft but not brown.
2. Sprinkle the flour over the vegetables, and stir until well combined. Keep cooking over medium heat for 2 to 3 minutes, until the flour begins to give off a nutty aroma.
3. Add the wine, stock, salt, saffron, thyme, and bay leaf. Scrape up any flour that sticks to the bottom of the pot until all is incorporated. Bring to a boil and simmer, covered, for about 15 minutes. Remove and discard the bay leaf.
4. Add 20 shrimp, and simmer for 2 to 3 minutes more until they turn reddish pink. Puree the soup coarsely with an immersion blender, or transfer in batches to a blender or food processor, puree, and return to the pot. Simmer for 1 minute, and adjust the seasoning.
5. In a separate small pot, steam the 4 remaining shrimp in 1 inch of water until they turn reddish pink, 2 to 3 minutes. Serve the soup hot, garnished with a cooked shrimp and 1/2 teaspoon chives. Pass the pepper mill.

Makes about 4 servings

Shrimp Potage

3   shallots, minced
3   garlic cloves, minced
2   tablespoons extra virgin olive oil
1   tablespoon whole wheat flour
2   cups shrimp stock
1/2   teaspoon sea salt, or to taste
12   shrimp, peeled
1/8   teaspoon freshly ground white pepper, or to taste (optional)
1   teaspoon chopped fresh parsley, or greens of 1 scallion, sliced
        thinly on the diagonal

1. In a 2-quart pot, sauté the shallots and garlic in the oil over medium
   heat for 2 to 3 minutes, until translucent but not brown. Sprinkle the
   flour over the mixture, and stir until well blended.
2. Add the stock and salt, stirring with a wooden spoon until all is well
   blended. Simmer for 10 minutes.
3. Add the shrimp, and simmer for 2 to 3 minutes until they turn reddish
   pink. Puree the soup coarsely with an immersion blender or in batches
   in a blender or food processor. Stir in the pepper, if using. Serve hot,
   garnished with the chopped parsley or sliced scallions.

Makes 2 servings

5-Hour Whole Fish Soup

This soup is a variation on a classic Japanese carp soup called Koi Ko Ku, which is traditionally recommended as a tonic and blood strengthener for women who have given birth. Because of the long cooking, the fish bones are completely softened and become edible and quite delicious. It is a superior source of natural calcium and other essential bone minerals: in fact, 1 cup provides more than 800 mg of calcium.

1   whole fish (e.g., pike, red snapper, carp), about 1^1/$_2$ to
      2 pounds
4   slices ginger
3   small carrots (about ^{1}/$_2$ pound), scrubbed and cut into chunks
1   medium onion, cut into medium dice
1   cup white wine or ^{1}/$_4$ cup brown rice vinegar
6   cups water
^{1}/$_4$ cup mellow barley miso

1. Buy only very fresh fish. Ask your fishmonger to clean it, leaving on the scales, head, and tail, and cut it into 3 to 4 pieces. Rinse well before cooking.
2. Cut 4 thin slices off a piece of gingerroot, lay them on top of each other, and slice them lengthwise into thin slivers.
3. Place the fish, ginger, carrots, onion, wine, water, and miso in a 6-quart pressure cooker. Bring up to pressure, reduce the heat to low, and simmer very gently for 5 hours. Allow to sit until the pressure is down, open the pot, and stir vigorously with a wooden spoon to blend the flavors. Check the amount of liquid: it should be soupy, not too dry; add some water if needed. Test a bone; it should be easy to chew. If a little too hard, pressure-cook for another hour. This soup can be kept in the refrigerator for 4 days. I do not recommend freezing because it kills the taste and makes it flat. Reboil each time before serving, adding a little stock or water if necessary.

Makes 6 to 8 servings

Sunflower Seed Soup

1 onion, coarsely diced (about 1 cup)
2 carrots, cut into chunks (about 2 cups)
1 celery root (celeriac), peeled, cut into medium dice (about
     2 cups)
1 small turnip, diced (about 3/4 cup)
4 cups vegetable stock
1/2 cup raw sunflower seeds
1 teaspoon sea salt, or to taste
1 teaspoon umeboshi vinegar, or 1 teaspoon lemon juice and a
     pinch of salt
1 tablespoon grated fresh ginger
2 teaspoons chopped fresh tarragon

1. Place the onion, carrots, celery root, turnip, stock, sunflower seeds, and
   salt in a 4-quart pot. Bring to a boil, lower the heat, cover, and simmer
   for 25 to 30 minutes, until all the vegetables are soft.
2. Puree in batches in a blender until creamy. Return to the pot. Bring
   back to a simmer, taste, and adjust the seasoning. Stir in the umeboshi
   vinegar or lemon juice and salt, the fresh ginger and tarragon, and serve
   hot. This soup thickens as it stands; dilute with water or stock as
   needed.

Makes 4 servings

Salads

A salad can be a great addition to a good meal, or it can be a meal in itself with the addition of some protein foods such as beans, chicken, or seafood. Salads are an easy way to bring vegetables and leafy greens into the diet, and the dressing can be a fine source of essential fatty acids.

Chickpea Tabbouleh

Chickpeas are delicious and lend themselves to many dishes, both cold and hot. They take a long time to cook, so I always use a pressure cooker. If they are old and very dry, they sometimes don't ever get soft in a regular pot, no matter how long you cook them, but I have found the pressure cooker always works. The dressing in this recipe is very mild; for a more sour, "salad-y" flavor, use a regular vinaigrette. This dish is great for a picnic or summer lunch, with some fresh corn on the cob.

1	cup dried chickpeas, picked over and rinsed
4	cups water or vegetable stock
1	piece kombu seaweed (about 4 inches)
1/2	teaspoon sea salt
1	medium onion, cut into small dice (about 1 cup)
1	cup minced parsley

Lemon Dressing

1 1/2	tablespoons lemon juice
1 1/2	tablespoons extra virgin olive oil
1 1/2	tablespoons flaxseed oil
1	teaspoon umeboshi vinegar (optional)

1. Soak the chickpeas overnight and drain. Place in a pressure cooker with the water, kombu, and salt, and cook under pressure for 45 minutes, or until soft. Turn off the heat, and allow the pressure to fall naturally before removing the cover.
2. Place the onion in a large serving bowl. Using a mesh strainer, remove the chickpeas from the water, leaving the kombu behind, drain, and add them to the onions while still hot.

3. Remove the kombu with the mesh strainer, tear it with a fork or knife (it should disintegrate easily), and add to the chickpeas. Reserve the cooking water for your next soup.

4. Prepare the dressing by mixing all the ingredients in a separate bowl. Pour over the chickpeas. With a fork, mix the chickpeas, dressing, and onion until well combined. Allow to cool to room temperature, add the parsley, and toss. Serve immediately, or store in the refrigerator until ready to serve. This salad keeps well for 5 to 6 days.

Makes about 4 to 6 servings

Cucumber and Radish Salad with Wakame and Walnut-Lime Dressing

This cool and refreshing salad is great for summertime eating.

1	ounce dried wakame seaweed, soaked 20 minutes
2	large cucumbers (about 6 inches each), peeled and cut lengthwise, seeds removed
6	large red radishes
2	tablespoons lime juice
2	tablespoons walnut oil
1	tablespoon flaxseed oil
1/4	teaspoon sea salt

1. Drain the wakame, cut away the tough middle rib, and chop the leaves very fine. Place in a salad bowl.
2. Slice the cucumbers crosswise into 1/4-inch slices. Add to the bowl.
3. Scrub the radishes well. Cut them into quarters so that the red shows. Add to the bowl.
4. Whisk together the lime juice, walnut and flaxseed oils, and salt, and pour over the vegetables, tossing thoroughly. Marinate for at least 1 hour.

Makes 4 to 6 servings

Composed Salad with Beets and Avocado

2 large beets, unpeeled, with 1-inch stem and uncut root
1/4 pound (about 4 cups) mesclun or spring greens salad mix
1 ripe Haas avocado
Creamy Lemon-Ginger Dressing (see below)

1. Cook the beets in water to cover for about 1 hour, or until a sharp knife pierces them easily. Cool, peel with your hands under running cold water, and cut in half top to bottom. Slice into thin half-moons and set aside.
2. Divide the greens among 4 salad plates.
3. Cut the avocado in half lengthwise, and remove the pit. (Hint: Drop your knife into the avocado as if to cut the pit in half, so that the knife gets stuck in the pit, then twist gently, remove the pit on the knife, and discard.) Cut into quarters, and remove the peel. Slice each quarter into three thin lengthwise slices and fan on the greens.
4. Arrange the slices from half a beet on each plate. Drizzle about 1 tablespoon dressing over each serving of the beets and greens, and serve immediately.

Makes 4 servings

Creamy Lemon-Ginger Dressing

2 teaspoons ginger juice
3 tablespoons fresh lemon juice
3 tablespoons olive oil
3 tablespoons flaxseed oil
2 tablespoons water
2 tablespoons chopped scallions (white parts only)
1 teaspoon sea salt
4 ounces soft tofu (not silken)

Place all the ingredients in a blender and blend until smooth and creamy.

Mixed Green Salad

This standard salad is always pleasing, and goes with everything.

4   cups mixed baby greens or mesclun, loosely packed
1   tablespoon extra virgin olive oil
1   tablespoon flaxseed oil
1   tablespoon fresh lemon juice
1   teaspoon umeboshi vinegar, or $1/8$ teaspoon sea salt
1   teaspoon mustard
1   Belgian endive, sliced crosswise into $1/2$-inch slices

1. Place the greens in a serving bowl.
2. Place the oils, lemon juice, vinegar, and mustard in a small bowl or jar, and whisk or shake until well mixed. Toss the greens with the dressing.
3. Serve and sprinkle the Belgian endive slices over each portion.

Makes 4 servings

Fresh Fruit Salad with Toasted Sunflower Seeds

This dish is in the salad section because of its name, but it can just as easily be a dessert or even a breakfast. It is a good way to use fruit that is beginning to get too soft. Any fruit you have on hand can be used in a salad, although I avoid using melons or watermelons because some people like myself feel better when eating melon alone on an empty stomach, rather than mixed with other fruits. The juice oozing out of the orange wedges will help keep the apple from turning brown. The banana lends a lovely, soft, sweet flavor to contrast with the liveliness of the other fruits. Try to use organic fruits: they taste wonderful.

2   oranges, peeled and sectioned
2   apples, peeled if not organic, cored, and cut into 8 wedges
1   banana, thinly sliced
1   cup seedless green grapes
1/2   pint raspberries or strawberries
1   cup apple or orange juice
1   cup toasted sunflower seeds

Cut the orange and apple sections crosswise twice, so that each wedge yields three pieces. Place in a large bowl. Add the rest of the ingredients, toss, and serve. Keeps for 1 day.

Makes 4 servings

Vegetables from Land and Sea

Everybody should eat more vegetables. Current recommendations are five to seven servings per day. This can be done with soup, salad, and side dishes at lunch and dinner, even breakfast. If there is no time for soup at lunch, then snacking on raw veggies is always an option. I often eat greens with my hot breakfast.

You can find fresh vegetables at supermarkets, health food stores, vegetable stands, and green markets. Summer vegetables, such as asparagus, zucchini, yellow squash, and snow peas, are quick cooking and easy to prepare. Winter vegetables, such as turnips and rutabaga, are great in soups and stews.

Greens need to be part of every healthful eating style. They are an essential source of calcium and other nutrients such as iron and vitamin A. Most people ignore these important foods, because, as Rudolph Ballantine, M.D., has pointed out in his book *Diet and Nutrition*, the modern preparation method of steaming instead of boiling leaves them tough and bitter. Strong-tasting greens, which are very important for our bone health, should always be boiled for fifteen to twenty minutes, and then prepared as desired for the dish. The boiling removes the bitter taste and makes the greens softer and sweeter. Even when boiled, dark leafy greens are high in nutrients: one cup of boiled, drained greens contains about 100 percent of the RDA for vitamin C, 100 percent of the RDA for vitamin A, and between 10 and 20 percent of the RDA for calcium and iron.

Asparagus with Slivered Almonds

Asparagus are quick and easy to prepare, and everyone loves them. They can be served hot, cold, or at room temperature.

  1   pound fresh asparagus
  1   cup boiling water or as needed
  1/4 cup blanched slivered almonds

1. Rinse the asparagus. Snap off the bottom half wherever it breaks and discard. Place enough asparagus in a large skillet to fit in one layer, pour boiling water over them to come up 1/2 inch, and cover.
2. Steam for 3 to 4 minutes. Repeat with remaining asparagus. Serve immediately with 1 tablespoon of almonds sprinkled on each serving.

Makes 4 servings

Basic Garlic Greens

This type of dish should be consumed almost daily for healthy bones. It is great as an accompaniment to a hot breakfast cereal, lunch, or dinner. A traditional way of preparing these greens would be to simmer them in a stock made by boiling a ham hock in 5 to 6 cups of water with 1 tablespoon of wine vinegar for 2 hours; using this stock would make the dish extra calcium-rich. Leftover greens can be beaten with an organic egg or two and made into a "green scramble."

1/2   pound kale, collards, or mustard greens
1   teaspoon extra virgin olive oil
2   garlic cloves, chopped
1   to 1 1/2 cups vegetable or chicken stock or water
      pinch of sea salt
      pinch of grated nutmeg

1. Cut the tough stems off the greens. Wash the leaves well and pat dry. Pile up, then cut lengthwise and crosswise into bite-size pieces.
2. In a large saucepan, heat the oil gently, add the garlic, stir for a minute, then add the greens and the stock. Push the greens under the liquid with a wooden spoon. Simmer, uncovered, for 15 to 20 minutes. Add the salt, grate a dusting of nutmeg over the greens, and stir for 2 minutes.

Makes about 4 servings

Cajun Kale with Carrots and Turnip

1   tablespoon extra virgin olive oil
1   medium onion, coarsely diced (about 1 cup)
1 to 3   teaspoons Cajun blackening seasoning
3   small carrots, cut into matchsticks (about 2 cups)
1   medium turnip, cut into large dice (about 2 cups)
2   cups vegetable stock
1/2   teaspoon sea salt
1   bunch kale or turnip greens, stems removed, cut into bite-size
      pieces (about 4 cups)

1. In a 4-quart saucepan, heat the oil and sauté the onion for about 2 min-utes, until translucent. Add the Cajun seasoning (1 teaspoon is mild, 3 is strong) and stir for another minute or two.
2. Add the carrots and turnip, and sauté for about 1 minute. Then add the stock and salt. Stir well to scrape up all browned bits from the bottom of the pot. Simmer, covered, for 20 minutes.
3. Uncover and add the greens, pushing them under the liquid and turn-ing the vegetables. The kale will shrink and soften and mix between the carrots and turnips. Keep simmering over low heat, uncovered, stirring once or twice, for another 15 minutes. Serve hot as a side dish.

Makes 4 to 6 servings

Stir-fried Bok Choy with Shrimp

For a vegetarian variation, replace the shrimp with cubed, seasoned, smoked tofu (available in health food stores).

 4 leaves bok choy, whites and greens
 2 large garlic cloves, minced
 2 thin slices fresh ginger, minced
 2 whole scallions, whites and greens, thinly sliced
 1 tablespoon extra virgin olive oil
 2 tablespoons natural soy sauce (shoyu or tamari)
 2 tablespoons water or shrimp stock
12 medium shrimp, peeled

1. Wash the bok choy leaves well. Cut off and discard a 1-inch slice from the bottom to get rid of the root and loosen the stems. Cut off the greens along the thick white stem. Cut the whites once lengthwise, then crosswise into 1/2-inch pieces. Pile up the greens, cut twice lengthwise, then cut them across into 1- to 2-inch pieces. Prep the rest of the vegetables.

2. Heat a wok or a 3- to 4-quart pot, add the oil, then the garlic, ginger, and scallions. Stir with a wok spatula or wooden spoon over medium-high heat. Add the whites of the bok choy, and stir for another 1 to 2 minutes. Sprinkle 1 tablespoon of the soy sauce and the stock over the whites. Lower the heat to low, place a cover over the wok or pot, and allow to cook for 6 to 8 minutes.

3. Uncover, raise the heat to medium-high, add the greens, and stir for a minute or two until they're wilted. Add the shrimp, and sprinkle with the remaining tablespoon of soy sauce. Stir for 2 to 4 minutes, until the shrimp firm, curl up, and become reddish pink. Serve immediately.

Makes 2 to 3 servings

Broccoli Rabe with Roasted Garlic and Red Pepper

This dish can take the place of salad; it keeps well for 3 days.

1   head garlic, cloves separated but unpeeled
1   tablespoon plus 1 teaspoon extra virgin olive oil
1   bunch broccoli rabe (about 1 pound)
4   cups water
1   large red pepper
1   tablespoon flaxseed oil
1   tablespoon lemon juice

1. Preheat the oven to 400 degrees F. Rub the garlic cloves with 1 teaspoon olive oil, place on a baking sheet, and roast in the oven for 20 to 25 minutes, or until soft but not burned. Peel and set aside.
2. While the garlic cooks, prepare the broccoli rabe. Cut off the tough stems, wash the leaves well, and pat dry. Chop coarsely into bite-size pieces.
3. Heat the water or stock in a 4-quart pot, add the broccoli rabe, and put a plate on top of the greens to keep them under water. Simmer for 15 to 20 minutes. Drain. (You can drink a cup of the "pot likker," or what my children used to call "greens' water," with a dash of lemon juice or umeboshi vinegar for an excellent mineral-rich tonic. Do not keep this cooking water, as it turns very bitter once it cools.)
4. Roast the red pepper by placing it directly on the trivet of the gas flame, or under the broiler or in a 400-degree F oven. Turn it with tongs until it is black and charred all over. Place it in a small pot and cover, or in a brown paper bag, to sweat and loosen the skin. After 20 minutes, wash under running water to remove all the charred skin. (This leaves a flavorful, bright red "pimento," which can be used as a colorful garnish in many dishes.) Cut lengthwise into strips, discarding the seeds and top, then across into squares.
5. Mix the remaining 1 tablespoon olive oil, the flaxseed oil, and the lemon juice. Toss the broccoli rabe with the peeled garlic cloves, red pepper squares, and olive oil mix. Serve at room temperature.

Makes about 4 servings

Curried Mustard Greens with Parmesan

This delicious dish is a combination of Indian and Italian ideas.

1	bunch mustard greens or broccoli rabe (about 1 pound)
2	tablespoons clarified butter (Ghee, *see* page 114) or extra virgin olive oil
3	large garlic cloves, thinly sliced
1	tablespoon curry powder
1/4	teaspoon sea salt
1/4	cup grated Parmesan cheese

1. Cut off most of the thick stems of the greens. Wash well in several changes of water. Place in a 4-quart saucepan with about 2 cups water, push under, and cook for 8 to 10 minutes, or until bright green and soft. Remove from the pot and chop into bite-size pieces. Discard the cooking water or drink a cup as described in Broccoli Rabe recipe.
2. In a 10-inch skillet, heat the clarified butter or oil, add the garlic slices, and sauté until they begin to brown lightly. Add the curry powder and mix well, then add the salt. Add the chopped greens and mix well; heat for 5 to 8 minutes, stirring often.
3. Sprinkle the Parmesan over all, mix, and serve.

Makes about 4 servings

Gingered Kale with Miso-broiled Tofu

This is a flexible recipe. You can make it as is, or you can make just the greens or just the tofu. You can use mustard or collard greens instead of the kale. The water left over from cooking the greens is nutritive and delicious if you add a bit of lemon juice or umeboshi vinegar; have a cup while you cook the rest of your meal. The tofu can be served on its own as a snack or appetizer.

> 1 pound kale, tough stems removed, washed (about 5 cups)
> 3 cups water
> 8 thin slices fresh ginger
>   Miso-broiled Tofu (see below)
> 1 tablespoon extra virgin olive oil

1. In a 4-quart soup pot, add the greens, water, and 4 slices of ginger. Simmer, uncovered, for about 15 minutes, using a wooden spoon to push the greens under the water. When done, fish out the greens and place them in a colander to drain. Chop coarsely and set aside.
2. Cut the broiled tofu into dice (once lengthwise and twice crosswise) and set aside. Mince the remaining slices of ginger.
3. Heat the oil in a skillet, and add the minced ginger, sautéing for 30 seconds. Add the chopped greens and diced tofu and stir well until hot, about 2–3 minutes. Serve immediately.

Makes 4 servings

Miso-broiled Tofu

> 12 ounces firm tofu
> 1 tablespoon organic mellow barley miso
> 1 teaspoon lemon juice
> 1/2 teaspoon prepared Dijon mustard
> 1 1/2 teaspoons extra virgin olive oil
> 1 tablespoon water

1. Slice the tofu into 8 1/2-inch slabs, and lay them flat in a shallow baking pan.
2. Mix the miso, lemon juice, mustard, oil, and water until they form a

thickish paste. Brush or smear over both sides of the tofu slices. Allow to sit for 15 to 20 minutes.

3. Broil about 5 minutes on each side, turning over once, or until nicely browned.

Broccoli with Mushrooms

Here is a delicious and simple way to prepare this popular vegetable.

2   broccoli stalks
1   tablespoon extra virgin olive oil
2   large garlic cloves, minced
4   ounces button mushrooms, sliced
1/4 teaspoon sea salt
1/4 cup water

1. Cut the florets off the broccoli stalks and place in a bowl. Peel the stalks with a vegetable peeler or sharp knife. Cut off the bottom 1/2 inch. Slice the stalks thinly on the diagonal and place in another bowl.
2. In a large skillet or wok, heat the oil over medium heat, add the garlic, and sauté for 10 seconds. Add the sliced mushrooms and sprinkle with salt. Stir and shake a bit until the mushrooms begin to release some liquid. Add the broccoli stems and mix well. Cover, lower the heat, and cook for 5 minutes.
3. Add the broccoli florets to the skillet and mix thoroughly. Add the water, cover, and cook for 5 to 6 minutes, or until the florets are a deep green. Serve immediately.

Makes 4 to 6 servings

Note: Sprinkle a little dark sesame oil over the broccoli just before serving, if you wish, for a real Chinese taste.

Baked Buttercup Squash

This cooking technique can be used with any hard winter squash or pumpkin, although cooking times might vary. Make soup with the leftovers by blending with sautéed onions and stock.

> 1   medium buttercup squash (the squat green one)
> 2   tablespoons vegetable stock
> 2   tablespoons butter, flaxseed oil, or olive oil, or to taste

1. Preheat the oven to 400 degrees F.
2. Scrub the squash well. Cut in half from stem to stem, brush the cut edges with a little olive oil, and place seed-side down, on a cookie sheet or baking pan lined with parchment paper. Bake in the preheated oven for about 1 to 1½ hours, depending on the size. The squash is done when it can be easily pierced through with a knife.
3. Remove the seeds with a spoon and discard. With a fork, mash the squash in the skin; moisten with a little stock, and add butter, flaxseed oil, or olive oil to taste. Spoon out of the skin onto individual plates as a side dish.

Makes about 4 servings

Butternut Squash with Onions and Tarragon

This is a delicious and easy way to make squash. If you have any leftovers, puree in the blender with enough stock or water to reach the consistency of cream soup; then reheat and season to taste with salt and pepper.

1   cup chopped onion (about 1 medium onion)
3   large garlic cloves, minced
1   tablespoon extra virgin olive oil
1/2 teaspoon dried tarragon
1   medium butternut squash, peeled and cut into large dice
1/2 teaspoon sea salt
1/2 cup vegetable or chicken stock or water, or enough to cover the
     bottom of the pan by 1/2 inch

1. In a 4-quart saucepan, sauté the onion and garlic in the oil for 1 to 2 minutes, or until translucent. Add the tarragon and mix.
2. Add the squash, mix well, and sprinkle with the salt. Add the stock or water, cover, and cook over very low heat for 25 to 30 minutes, or until the squash is soft. Serve hot.

Makes 4 servings

Puree of Yams

Here is an excellent way to get beta carotene and essential fatty acids into people who dislike healthy foods.

    2   medium yams (or sweet potatoes, the orange kind)
          (about 2/3 pounds)
    2   cups vegetable stock
  1/2   tablespoon unrefined flaxseed oil
    1   teaspoon butter

1. Peel the yams and cut into big chunks. Place them in a saucepan with the stock, which should come up about 1/2 inch from the bottom. Cover and simmer for about 30 minutes, or until soft. Strain the stock and set aside.
2. Mash the yams in the pot with a fork or potato masher, using enough stock (about 1/2 to 1 cup) to attain the consistency you like; add the flaxseed oil and butter, mixing well. Serve hot.

Makes about 3 cups, or 6 servings

Gratin of Root Vegetables

1   small rutabaga, peeled, cut in half lengthwise, and sliced into
     $1/2$-inch slices
1   sweet potato or yam, peeled and sliced into $1/2$-inch slices
2   small turnips, peeled and sliced into $1/2$-inch slices
1   medium parsnip, peeled and thinly sliced
2   tablespoons extra virgin olive oil
2   tablespoons whole wheat pastry flour
$2/3$ cup hot vegetable stock (optional)
$1/2$ teaspoon sea salt
     Freshly ground pepper
$1/4$ cup toasted whole wheat bread crumbs

1. Bring 6 cups of water to a boil, and blanch the rutabaga for 5 minutes. Add the rest of the vegetables, and blanch for another 5 minutes. Drain, reserving both the water and the vegetables.
2. Preheat the oven to 400 degrees F. Place the vegetables in an oiled ovenproof casserole, overlapping the slices.
3. To make a roux, heat the oil in a 1-quart saucepan, add the flour, and stir for 3 to 4 minutes until fragrant and lightly browned. Whisk in $2/3$ cup hot stock, if using, or reserved vegetable blanching water, and stir well to eliminate all lumps. Bring to a boil while continuously stirring. Add the salt, lower the heat to minimum, cover, and cook for about 10 minutes. Taste and add salt and pepper as desired.
4. Pour the sauce over the vegetables, cover, and bake for about 35 minutes. Uncover, sprinkle with bread crumbs, and bake another 25 minutes.

Makes about 6 servings

French Tart with Greens and Leeks

This tart is excellent for using up leftover greens, broccoli, and the like. Take it on a picnic! It was inspired by a recipe from Patricia Wells's Bistro Cooking.

Pastry

1/2 cup brown rice flour
1/2 cup whole wheat pastry flour
1/2 teaspoon sea salt
1/4 cup water
1/4 cup extra virgin olive oil

Filling

3 cups leeks, white and tender green parts, cleaned and sliced (see page 102)
1/2 cup water
1 cup leftover cooked or stir-fried greens (broccoli, bok choy, kale, etc.)
3 extra large organic eggs
1/2 cup freshly grated Parmesan cheese

1. Preheat the oven to 350 degrees F. To make the pastry, mix the flours and salt in a bowl until well blended. Add the oil, and stir with a wooden spoon to make medium pebbles. Add the water, and stir until it begins to hang together. Knead briefly in the bowl to obtain a moist dough. Press into a 10-inch pie plate to make an evenly thick crust all around; smooth out the borders. Prebake for 10 to 12 minutes and remove from the oven.
2. To make the filling, steam the cleaned and chopped leeks in the water for 4 minutes. Drain and place in a bowl. Add the leftover cooked greens and mix well.
3. Crack the eggs into a bowl and beat for about 30 seconds, then add the Parmesan. Pour over the greens and mix with a wooden spoon. Pour all into the prebaked pie crust, and return to the oven for 35 to 40 minutes, or until the eggs are firm.

Makes 6 servings

Gingered Vegetable Caviar with
Tofu and Dried Mushrooms

This is a powerful side dish; use only 2 or 3 tablespoons per person. It keeps well for a week, and can also be served cold as a topping for a green salad or even in a sandwich.

1/2	cup dried hiziki (hijiki) seaweed
1/4	cup each dried porcini and shiitake mushrooms, soaked in 2 cups warm water
1	tablespoon unrefined sesame oil
1	tablespoon minced garlic
1	tablespoon minced ginger
1 to 2	tablespoons natural soy sauce (shoyu or tamari)
8	ounces firm tofu, cubed

1. Place the hiziki in a paper bag and crush with a rolling pin. Soak in 2 cups water for 30 to 40 minutes. Drain, discarding the water. Chop very fine.
2. Drain the mushrooms, reserving the soaking liquid. Cut off the stems and discard; chop the mushrooms coarsely.
3. In a large skillet, heat the sesame oil, add the garlic and ginger, stir for 15 seconds, then add the chopped hiziki. Sauté for 1 minute. Add the mushrooms, soy sauce, and tofu. Pour in the mushroom soaking water, leaving gritty residue behind. Cook over low heat for 15 to 20 minutes, uncovered, until the liquid has almost evaporated.

Makes 6 servings

Whole Grains

Whole grains (brown rice, barley, oats, whole wheat, rye, quinoa, millet, buckwheat, and others) are those cereal grains that have the germ, the bran, and the starch intact as nature made them. When whole (not ground up) they can be planted or sprouted, and new shoots will emerge, showing how full of life they are. Refined grain, on the other hand, is missing both the bran and the germ and therefore the B vitamins, fiber, minerals, and vitamin E, and obviously does not sprout.

Because of their protective bran covering, whole grains are hard to digest; they need to be cooked well to become soft and digestible. For maximum digestibility, they can be soaked for about eight hours in water to cover by about one inch with a teaspoon of something sour, such as lemon, apple cider vinegar, umeboshi vinegar, or yogurt. Discard the water, and cook the grains with fresh water. The soaking inactivates the phytates present in the bran, which can interfere with the absorption of minerals such as iron, calcium, magnesium, and zinc.

Remember, whole grains should be well chewed to aid digestion!

Flavorful Rice and Barley

This is the basic cooking technique for whole grains such as brown rice, barley, millet, and quinoa.

- 1/2 cup brown rice
- 1/2 cup barley
- 2 cups filtered or spring water
- 1 tablespoon sauerkraut liquid, umeboshi vinegar, or organic yogurt
- 2 cups vegetable or chicken stock
- 1 bay leaf
  pinch of dried oregano
- 1/2 teaspoon sea salt, or to taste

1. Place the rice and barley in a bowl, add cold tap water, swirl around well to loosen all the dirt, and pour off the dirty water carefully, catching the grain in a colander. Repeat if necessary until the water runs clean.
2. Add 2 cups of water and the sauerkraut liquid, umeboshi vinegar, or yogurt to the grain, and let soak overnight. Drain before cooking.

3. When ready to cook, place the drained grain in a 2- or 3-quart sauce-pan, add the stock, bay leaf, oregano, and salt, bring to a boil, and simmer without stirring, covered, for 1 hour. For a fluffier grain, add the stock boiling hot.

Makes about 4 servings

Creamy Millet Breakfast Porridge

This excellent breakfast dish is hearty and satisfying. If you have leftovers, keep them in the fridge and reheat by steaming in a small pot with 1/4 cup water per portion. Omit the nuts if you have a tendency to pimples or acne. Add a side of sauerkraut or cooked greens for some extra calcium. You can also try a mixture of two grains: barley and rice, or millet and quinoa.

1   cup millet
7   cups filtered water
1   teaspoon fresh lemon juice, or 2 teaspoons umeboshi vinegar
      or natural sauerkraut liquid
1   teaspoon sea salt
4   tablespoons raw almonds
4   tablespoons roasted sunflower seeds
4   tablespoons flaxseed oil
4   teaspoons natural soy sauce or 4 teaspoons maple syrup
      (optional)

1. At night, wash and drain the grain. Place in a 2-quart saucepan with 2 cups of the water and 1 teaspoon of the lemon juice, umeboshi vinegar, or sauerkraut liquid. Cover and soak overnight.
2. In the morning, drain the grain. Add the remaining 5 cups of water and the salt to the grain, bring to a boil, then lower the heat and simmer, covered, for about 1 hour and 15 minutes, without stirring.
3. Place a portion (about 1 cup) in each of 4 soup plates. Divide almonds, sunflower seeds, and flaxseed oil, and add to each serving; season with soy sauce or maple syrup, stir well, and enjoy.

Makes 4 servings

Plain Kasha

This is easy and quick to make, and goes well as a starch with many dishes. Kasha is a warming food, excellent for cooler weather. It also tastes less acid-forming than other grains, probably because it's technically not really a grain but a grass. To reheat, steam in 1/4 inch of water or stock.

2¹/₂ cups vegetable stock
¹/₄ teaspoon sea salt
1 cup whole kasha (roasted buckwheat)

In a 1-quart saucepan, bring the stock and salt to a boil. Add the kasha, lower the heat, cover, and simmer for about 15 minutes.

Makes 5 to 6 servings

Kasha with Mushrooms

This side dish is excellent for winter meals. Try it with some Parsley Sauce (page 159), Baked Buttercup Squash (page 140), and Simple Roast Chicken (page 164).

    1/2   cup dried porcini mushrooms, soaked in 2 cups warm water
          or vegetable or chicken stock
      1   cup kasha (roasted buckwheat)
    1/4   cup sunflower seeds
    1/2   teaspoon sea salt

1. Soak the mushrooms for 30 minutes. Drain, reserving the soaking water. Chop the mushrooms coarsely.
2. Measure the soaking water leaving the gritty residue behind, and add enough water or vegetable or chicken stock to make 2 cups of liquid. Pour into a 2-quart saucepan and bring to a boil.
3. Add the kasha, sunflower seeds, mushrooms, and salt to the boiling liquid. Lower the heat to a simmer, cover, and cook for 15 minutes, or until the grain is fluffy. Mix with a fork. Serve hot.

Makes about 4 servings

Polenta

For a variation on this great side dish, use olive oil instead of butter and stir in 1/2 cup black Greek olives just before serving.

  2^1/$_2$ cups vegetable or chicken stock
   ^{1}/$_4$ teaspoon sea salt
   ^{1}/$_2$ cup yellow corn grits or polenta (coarse grind)
  1   tablespoon butter

1. Bring the stock to a boil with the salt. Whisk in the polenta, stirring continuously until it has thickened. Keep over low heat, and stir for 3 to 4 minutes, then cover and cook for 8 to 10 minutes or according to package directions. Stir in the butter.
2. Polenta is mushy at first, but stiffens as it cools. Here are several serving suggestions: serve straight out of the pot onto a plate; pour into a bowl, let it firm up for about 15 minutes, turn onto a plate, and cut using a string stretched between your hands; pour into individual serving bowls or cups, then turn onto individual plates after it firms up; make more than you need, keep the leftovers in a loaf pan, then slice and fry for breakfast.

Makes about 2 servings

Rice and Millet Pilaf with Almonds and Cilantro

1/2	cup long-grain brown rice
1/2	cup millet
1	teaspoon olive oil
1	teaspoon cumin
1	teaspoon turmeric
2¹/4	cups boiling chicken or vegetable stock
1/2	teaspoon sea salt
1/4	cup blanched almonds, coarsely chopped
2	tablespoons cilantro, finely chopped
2	scallions, thinly sliced

1. To wash each grain well, put in a bowl, add cold water, swirl it around, and pour off the dirty water. (If desired, soak grain overnight as per page 146.) Then pour the grain into a colander.
2. Heat the oil in a 4-quart saucepan, add the spices, cook for 10 seconds, then add the grain. Stir over medium heat for 4 to 5 minutes. Add the boiling stock, the salt, stir once or twice, and bring to a boil. Lower the heat to low, cover, and cook for 45 to 50 minutes, or until fluffy.
3. Prepare the almonds, cilantro, and scallions. Stir into the pilaf just before serving.

Makes about 6 servings

Oat-Dulse Crackers

These crackers made from a traditional Irish recipe are delicious with any hearty soup and keep well, too. To make them more cookielike, use butter instead of oil, and add 1/2 teaspoon of baking powder to the flour mixture. If you don't like the seaweed taste, use agar flakes instead of the dulse; agar is just as high in nutrients but has a very mild taste.

　　2　cups oatmeal or rolled oats
　　1　cup sunflower seeds
　1/2　cup whole wheat pastry flour
　　4　tablespoons dulse flakes (see Note)
　1/2　teaspoon sea salt
　1/3　cup canola oil or melted butter
　　1　cup water
　　1　teaspoon caraway or toasted sesame seeds (optional)

1. Grind the oatmeal and sunflower seeds separately in a food processor. Pour both into a large bowl with the pastry flour and the dulse flakes, and mix well with a fork.
2. Add the salt, oil or butter, and water to a separate bowl; whisk briefly to blend, then add to the oatmeal mixture. Stir well with a wooden spoon until all the oats are moistened. The mixture should be the texture of thick tuna salad. Cover and let stand 8 hours or overnight.
3. Preheat the oven to 350 degrees F. Line a large metal baking pan with parchment paper. Place tablespoonfuls of the oat mixture on the parchment paper and press down with the back of a fork to make 1/2-inch-thick rounds. Sprinkle a few seeds, if using, over the top and press down with the fork. Bake for 20 to 25 minutes, until browned around the edges, dry, and crisp.

Makes about sixteen 3-inch crackers; 1 serving is 2 crackers

Note: Dulse flakes can be found in natural food stores as a condiment.

Beans

Beans or legumes, a popular food in many cultures, are a fine source of vegetable protein, and should be eaten frequently by those who are vegetarians or semivegetarians. There are many different varieties available in our marketplace: lentils, split peas, kidney beans, navy beans, pinto beans, black beans, chickpeas or garbanzos, and so many others.

Just like whole grains, beans need to be soaked to eliminate the phytates and especially to help break down the acids that cause gas. Always discard the soaking water and cook with fresh water to make beans more digestible. If you forget to soak the beans you are planning to use, you can do a quick soak if you have the time: bring the beans and soaking water to a boil, simmer for two or three minutes, turn off the heat, and let sit, covered, for about two hours. Discard the water. Legumes go well with spices such as curries or cumin, which help digestibility.

It may be more efficient to make one pot of plain cooked legumes, and then use them in other dishes (soups, stews, salads) that will, in turn, need less cooking time.

Remember to chew your beans well!

Root Stew with White Beans and Chanterelles

This is a great winter stew; it's best to make a lot, as it keeps well in the refrigerator for several days. Should you get bored with the same taste, add some extra stock to the last leftover servings and puree it all in the blender to make a creamy soup.

1/2   cup dried white beans, washed and soaked 8 hours in 4 cups
      water
2   bay leaves
1/4   cup dried chanterelles or other dried wild mushroom
2   tablespoons extra virgin olive oil
2   garlic cloves, minced
1   onion, coarsely diced
1   teaspoon dried thyme
1   teaspoon turmeric
2   carrots, cut into chunks

4-inch daikon (Japanese white radish), cut into chunks (about
   2 cups)
1   small yellow turnip or rutabaga, peeled and cut into chunks
      (about 3 cups)
1   burdock root, shaved (like a pencil) or julienned (optional)
1   cup water
1   cup vegetable stock
1/2   teaspoon sea salt, or to taste
4   teaspoons fresh chopped cilantro
4   teaspoons chopped scallions

1. Drain the beans, place them in a small pot with enough water to cover
   by 1 inch, add 1 bay leaf, and simmer for 1 hour while you prep the
   vegetables and proceed with the recipe.
2. Soak the dried mushrooms in 1 cup hot water for 20 minutes.
3. In a 6- to 8-quart pot, heat the oil over medium heat, add the garlic and
   onion, and stir for 2 minutes, or until translucent. Add the thyme and
   turmeric, stir, and add the carrots, daikon, turnip, and burdock.
4. Add the water, stock, and salt to the vegetable pot. Add the remaining
   bay leaf. The liquid should cover about two-thirds of the vegetables.
   Bring to a boil, lower the heat, and simmer for about 20 minutes.
5. Remove the mushrooms from the soaking water and slice thickly. Add
   to the vegetables along with the soaking water, pouring slowly so that
   any residual grit stays in the bowl. Simmer for 10 minutes.
6. Drain the beans, which should be 95 percent cooked, and add to the
   vegetables. Taste the liquid in the pot and add more salt if needed.
   Cover and simmer for 15 minutes. Remove bay leaf and discard. Serve
   with chopped cilantro and scallions.

Makes 8 to 10 servings

Anasazi Beans with Collards and Shiitake

Anasazi beans are reputed to be good at lowering cholesterol. They are delicious plain, with some fresh chopped parsley or cilantro; they are also excellent in soups and dips. The greens, of course, should be a staple. Try this dish with Rice and Millet Pilaf with Almonds and Cilantro (page 152) and some baked squash. Try a bowl for breakfast—after all, it's protein and calcium, just like milk!

1	cup dried anasazi beans, soaked 8 hours in cold water
1	bay leaf
1	tablespoon extra virgin olive oil
3	garlic cloves, minced
	pinch of dried thyme
4	large fresh shiitake mushrooms, stems removed, sliced
1^1/4	teaspoons salt
3	large collard greens, stem removed, cut into 2 × 2-inch pieces
1	cup water

1. Drain the beans, place in a 3-quart pot, add water to cover by 2 inches, the bay leaf, 1 teaspoon salt, and simmer, covered, for 45 minutes or until soft. Or you can pressure-cook for 10 to 15 minutes and allow the pressure to come down naturally.
2. In a separate pot, heat the oil, sauté the garlic for 1 minute, add the thyme and the mushrooms, sprinkle the remaining 1/4 teaspoon salt over them, and stir over medium heat for 2 to 3 minutes. Add the greens and stir; then add the water, which should just barely cover the greens. Simmer, uncovered, for about 15 minutes. Remove with a slotted spoon to serve.
3. There are two ways to eat this dish: place the beans on top of the greens on the plate, or add the drained beans to the greens and heat together for about 5 minutes.

Makes about 6 servings

Fish and Chicken

Small portions of these foods provide excellent nutrition, especially when the fish is wild and the chicken organically raised. Farm-raised fish sometimes have either very bland or off flavors; they may also be fed or dipped in antibiotics. Commercially raised fowl receive numerous antibiotics in their feed. I find it best to buy chicken from a butcher shop and fish from a fish store, rather than a supermarket. Fortunately, there are now many natural food supermarkets and stores around the country that carry naturally raised chicken and meats, so we have more choices. Local farms can also be a good source of natural foods. Use them within a day of purchase.

What You Can Do to Prevent Food Poisoning

When preparing animal foods, attend to careful hygiene.

1. To clean your hands: Wash well with abundant soap and dry with a clean towel or paper towels.
2. To sanitize cutting boards and counter surfaces: Prepare a solution of 3 teaspoons chlorine bleach (any brand) in one gallon of water, and use to wipe surfaces clean. Do not rinse, just allow to air-dry. *Always* sanitize plates or cutting boards immediately after using them for raw meat, fish, chicken or any other animal foods, before you put any other food on them. To be even safer, cut meat, fish, chicken, or other animal foods on wax or parchment paper (perhaps the paper it came in), which can then be discarded. To clean wood cutting boards (which should never be immersed in water), saturate a sponge with white vinegar and wipe clean. To remove food particles from a wood board without using caustic chemicals that could get into the food, sprinkle the board with coarse salt or baking soda, and wipe clean with a damp cloth or sponge. Studies have shown that bacteria die quicker on wood than on plastic cutting boards.
3. To sanitize utensils: Wipe or immerse them in the same solution used to clean cutting boards and counter surfaces, or immerse in hot water (at least 170 degrees F) for a minimum of thirty seconds. A good dishwasher will normally reach these temperatures. Plastic cutting boards can also be placed in the dishwasher.
4. Wipe up spills of the juices of raw meat, fish, seafood, or chicken immediately, and sanitize the surfaces they fell on.
5. Wash your hands with soap again immediately after handling animal foods.

Crispy Baked Small Fish

This way of preparing small fish makes it easy to consume the bones. With this technique, only 1/2 cup of oil is used, instead of the usual 2 to 4 cups used in deep-frying. I had this dish analyzed for calcium, magnesium, potassium, sodium, and zinc. It also has small quantities of protein, a small amount of fat (from the olive oil), some carbohydrates from the cornmeal, and other minerals in the bones that were not analyzed. There was no equivalent food in the nutrition analysis software program, so I have no information on the rest of the nutrients. The incredible mineral richness of this recipe is clear in the nutrient chart in the Appendix. A little goes a long way!

1	pound fresh small whole fish, such as anchovies, smelts, or whitebait
1/2	cup cornmeal
1/2	teaspoon sea salt
1/2	teaspoon pepper
1/2	cup olive oil
4 to 6	lime or lemon wedges

1. Have the fish cleaned, but leave the heads and tails on.
2. Preheat the oven to 400 degrees F. Wash the fish in several changes of water until the water runs clear. Pat dry with paper towels.
3. Place the cornmeal, salt, and pepper in a plastic or paper bag and shake until mixed. Add the fish to the bag, and shake well until all the fish is covered. Put the olive oil in a soup plate, and dip the fish in it briefly.
4. Put the fish in a single layer in a large metal baking pan. (You can put some parchment paper in the pan to protect it.) Bake in the preheated oven for 30 to 40 minutes, depending on the size of the fish (whitebait takes only 20 minutes, larger smelts may take 40 to 45), until they are crisp and dry but not overbrowned. If the fish are longer than 3 1/2 inches, turn them over once about halfway through the cooking time. Serve hot or warm as an entrée, appetizer, or snack with 1 lime or lemon wedge per person.

Makes 3 to 4 servings

Poached Red Snapper Fillets with Parsley Sauce

Purchase a whole red snapper and have it filleted; take home both the fillets and the bones. To poach these delicate fillets, use fish stock from your freezer, or make some from the snapper's bones and trimmings. These fillets should be served warm, so make them just before serving.

    2   cups fish stock
    1   teaspoon dried rosemary
  1/2   teaspoon dried thyme
    4   cardamom pods
  1/4   teaspoon sea salt
    2   red snapper fillets

1. Place the fish stock in a large nonreactive skillet or poacher. Place the rosemary, thyme, and cardamom in a piece of 100 percent cotton cheesecloth and tie it well; hit it a few times with the handle of your knife or a big spoon to break up the spices slightly so they will release more flavor. Add this bouquet garni to the stock, as well as the salt. Heat to just below the boil.
2. Add the fillets to the skillet skin side up. Poach gently, never allowing the poaching liquid to boil, for about 5 minutes. Turn the fillets over, and continue poaching for another 3 to 4 minutes, depending on the thickness of the fillets. To test for doneness, push a knife through the fish; if it goes through easily, and the fish is white through and through, the poaching is done. Gently lift the fillets out of the poaching liquid; discard the bouquet garni, but keep the poaching liquid. Use some for the Parsley Sauce, add the rest to your fish stock stash.

Makes 2 servings

Parsley Sauce

    2   tablespoons clarified butter (*see* page 114)
    3   tablespoons whole wheat pastry flour
    1   cup hot fish poaching liquid or fish stock, or vegetable stock
  1/4   teaspoon sea salt, or to taste
    2   tablespoons minced fresh parsley
    1   teaspoon lemon juice
        freshly ground pepper

1. To make a roux, heat the clarified butter in a small saucepan over medium heat and add the flour. Stir with a wooden spoon continuously until the flour begins to brown very lightly and is fragrant. Whisk in the hot poaching liquid, stirring vigorously with a whisk first, then with a wooden spoon, until the mixture thickens and all lumps are worked out. Add the salt, and simmer covered over low heat for about 10 minutes, stirring occasionally. If too thick, add a little liquid.
2. Just before serving, remove from the heat and stir in the parsley and lemon juice. Grind fresh pepper into the sauce, and ladle over the fillets.

Makes about 1 cup

Salmon Omelet with Fresh Dill

This is great for a light lunch or hearty breakfast. For lunch, serve with Oat-Dulse Crackers (page 153) or whole-grain bread and a mixed green salad. For breakfast, replace the salad with brine-cured pickles or sauerkraut (the kind with no vinegar). It's good cold, too.

1	can (7.5 ounces) salmon, without oil or salt
1/4 to 1/2	teaspoon sea salt
2	teaspoons lemon juice
1	tablespoon chopped fresh dill, or 1 teaspoon dried oregano or basil
	freshly ground pepper
2	organic eggs
1	teaspoon unsalted or clarified butter (see page 114) or extra virgin olive oil

1. Drain the juice out of the can of salmon and put the rest of the contents in a mixing bowl. With a fork, mash the salmon well to break up all the pieces, skin, and bones. Add the salt, lemon juice, and dill, and mix well with the fork. Grind in the pepper to taste.
2. Break the eggs into the salmon mixture and mix in thoroughly.
3. Heat a 9-inch cast-iron or other type of skillet, and add the butter. Pour in the salmon-egg mixture and smooth out with the fork or a spatula. Cook over very low heat for 5 to 6 minutes, or until set. The whole omelet should slide around when you shake the pan. Turn over by sliding it onto a pot cover and turning it over into the pan, and cook another 3 minutes; you can also finish under the broiler.

Makes 2 servings

Sardine Spread

This is a terrific spread for crackers; use it as an appetizer or as part of a light lunch.

1	can (about 4³/₈ ounces) sardines, with skin and bones, packed in either oil or water
1	tablespoon fresh lemon juice
1	tablespoon grated onion
¹/₄	teaspoon sea salt
1	tablespoon tahini (unsalted sesame paste, optional)
1¹/₂	tablespoons chopped fresh parsley
4	rye crackers
	freshly ground pepper

Open the can of sardines partway, and drain out the oil or water. Place the sardines, lemon juice, onion, salt, tahini, and parsley in a bowl, and mash with a fork until well blended. Spread on whole rye crackers, and grind some pepper on top.

*Makes about 2 servings for lunch, or 8 when spread on
small crackers as an appetizer*

Crispy Chicken Wings

Chicken wings are an excellent potential source of calcium and other good bone minerals. The trick is to chew on the bone tips really well and eat as much of them as possible, including the marrow. The wings need to be well roasted, almost dry, for the bones to get soft and tasty. If you prefer to grill or barbecue the wings, a marinade for grilling follows.

> 2   pounds chicken wings
> salt and pepper to taste
> 2   tablespoons olive oil

1. Preheat the oven to 400 degrees F.
2. Wash the wings and pat dry. Rub with salt and pepper, and brush with a little olive oil. Bake for about 40 minutes, or until crisp.

Makes 4 servings

Marinade for Grilling

> 4   tablespoons natural soy sauce (shoyu or tamari)
> 2   tablespoons brown rice or wine vinegar
> 3   tablespoons extra virgin olive oil
> 2   teaspoons dried rosemary

In a small bowl, combine all the marinade ingredients; mix well. Place the chicken wings in a shallow pan, pour the rest of the marinade over them, and let sit for about 1 hour in the refrigerator. Turn over after 30 minutes. Grill or barbecue until crisp and brown.

Simple Roast Chicken

When you buy a chicken (always choose organic or free-range), keep the backbone, neck, and wing tips for stock. Then cut the rest of the chicken into 6 or 8 pieces, and roast as below. Freeze the carcass bones for stock as well. You can serve this with Polenta (page 151) and Cajun Kale with Carrots and Turnip (page 133).

1   organic chicken, cut up
1   tablespoon sea salt
1   teaspoon freshly ground pepper
1   teaspoon ground cumin
1/2   teaspoon ground ginger
1/2   cup chicken stock

1. Preheat the oven to 400 degrees F. Wash the chicken and pat it dry. Leave the skin on. Place skin side up in a large metal roasting pan lined with parchment paper.
2. In a small bowl or cup, blend the salt, pepper, cumin, and ginger. Rub the mixture all over the chicken pieces. Add about 1 cup water to the bottom of the pan. Bake for 45 to 60 minutes, or until the skin is crisp and the juices run clear when you poke a small knife into the largest piece.
3. Remove the chicken from the pan. Add a little hot chicken stock to the pan to pick up the brown bits and juices; pour it back into the stock stash or use as thin gravy over the chicken. Serve the chicken while still hot.

Makes 4 servings

What to Do with Leftover Cold Fish or Chicken

1. Add to any vegetable soup.
2. Add to a salad.
3. Put into a sandwich with whole-grain bread, salad greens, and a little salad dressing on the bread.
4. Stir-fry some vegetables, add fish or chicken pieces, and heat thoroughly.
5. Use as a quick snack with some celery and carrot sticks.

Desserts

For many people, dessert is the highlight of the meal. I do not belong to that group, so desserts I come up with are usually simple and don't take too long to make. I don't believe that desserts are really food unless they are made with whole-grain flours, fruit, and natural sweeteners. The recipes in this section are full of ingredients that are mineral-rich as well as high in essential fatty acids and fiber. Because they are too acid-forming, desserts made with white flour and white sugar are particularly detrimental to our health in general and promote rather than prevent osteoporosis.

For a sweet taste after a meal, the simpler and more natural the dessert, the better. In addition to these recipes, try dates, prunes, raisins, bananas, and natural applesauce with toasted almonds or sunflower seeds. Any fresh, seasonal fruit is, of course, an excellent choice.

Apple-Strawberry Mold

1³/4   cups apple-strawberry juice
¹/4   cup water
4   tablespoons agar (kanten) flakes
4   strawberries

1. Place the juice and water in a 2-quart saucepan and sprinkle the agar flakes over the surface. Bring to a gentle boil, and simmer for about 5 minutes, until the flakes have dissolved. Beat with a whisk to insure even dispersion.
2. Pour into a 2-cup mold and chill until set. To serve, unmold onto a plate and place the strawberries in the middle.

Makes 4 servings

Almond Milk Pudding

This is excellent either hot or cold!

2/3 cup blanched sliced almonds
2 1/4 cups filtered or spring water
1 teaspoon vanilla extract
1/3 cup kudzu powder
2 tablespoons maple syrup
　　 grated zest of 1/2 organic lemon
1/4 cup unsweetened apricot jam
2 tablespoons water
　　 chopped toasted almonds for garnish

1. Grind the blanched almonds in a coffee grinder until well powdered. Place in a blender with 1 1/2 cups of the water and blend for 1 to 2 minutes, until milky.
2. Place the almond mixture in a 1-quart saucepan with the vanilla extract. Simmer for 5 minutes. Strain through a fine strainer; place the leftover almond grounds back in the blender with 1/2 cup of the almond milk and blend again. Strain again. Return to the pot and bring back to a simmer.
3. In a small bowl, mix the kudzu with the remaining 3/4 cup water and the maple syrup and lemon zest until completely smooth. Add to the simmering almond milk, stirring vigorously until thickened and no lumps remain. Pour into four small ramekins. Mix the jam with the water, and spoon over the top of the pudding. Serve hot or cold, garnished with chopped toasted almonds.

Makes 4 servings

Broiled Bananas

This is a terrific quick-and-easy dessert. By the way, maple syrup has twice as much calcium as milk, ounce for ounce!

2   bananas, peeled, cut lengthwise and once crosswise
1   tablespoon clarified butter (see page 114)
1   tablespoon maple syrup
2   tablespoons water

1. Preheat the broiler. In a cast-iron skillet, sauté the bananas in the butter on one side only, for 2 to 3 minutes, or until soft and lightly browned.
2. Mix the maple syrup and water, and pour over the bananas. Place under the broiler for 2 to 3 minutes, or until the bananas begin to brown. Serve hot.

Makes 2 servings

Maple-Walnut Loaf

This rare treat is inspired by a recipe from one of the first natural foods cookbooks that I read, Beatrice Trum Hunter's Natural Foods Cookbook, *published in 1961. Because of the walnuts, it's an excellent source of omega-6 fatty acids.*

5	fresh whole organic eggs, separated
3/4	cup real maple syrup
1 1/2	cups walnuts, ground fine by pulsing in a food processor
1/2	cup whole wheat bread crumbs
	grated zest of 1 organic lemon (about 1/2 tablespoon)
	pinch each of ground cloves and mace
2	teaspoons vanilla extract

1. Preheat the oven to 325 degrees F. Line a 9 1/2-inch loaf pan with lightly buttered parchment paper.
2. In a large bowl, beat the egg yolks with the maple syrup for about 5 minutes, or until thick and frothy. Add the walnuts, bread crumbs, lemon zest, spices, and vanilla extract. Stir vigorously.
3. In a separate bowl (for best results, use a copper egg-beating bowl—you'll get much more volume), beat the whites with a whisk until they form almost firm peaks. (Lift the whisk and note how the egg whites stand up: If they bend over a lot, like a pointy cap drooping down, they're not ready. If they bend over just about 1/8 inch at the tip, they're ready. If they stand firm and straight up, they're overbeaten and run the risk of deflating fast.)
4. With a large rubber spatula, add a third of the beaten whites to the bowl with the yolk mixture. Fold in by turning over very gently from the outside inward. Do not stir! Repeat in thirds with the rest of the whites. You should have a very light, fluffy batter. Pour it into the prepared loaf pan, and bake without opening the oven door for about 1 hour and 20 minutes. The cake is done when a toothpick or thin knife inserted in the center comes out clean and dry. If not quite done, bake another 10 minutes.
5. Remove the loaf from the oven when ready, and invert over a cake rack covered with parchment paper. Peel off the paper. Cool. Slice and serve.

Makes 12 slices

Flax-Apple Shake

Thanks to D. Marcus Johnson, who helped me test all of these dishes, for this energizing recipe.

- 1/4 cup flaxseed, ground briefly in a coffee grinder
- 1   organic apple, cored, chopped into a few pieces
- 1/2 banana, sliced
- 2   cups unfiltered apple cider or juice

Place the flaxseed, apple, and banana in a blender, then add the apple cider or juice. Blend at low, then medium, speed until creamy. Drink immediately.

Makes 2 servings

Mineral-Rich Garnishes and Seasonings

Sesame Seaweed Sprinkle (Wakame Gomashio)

This recipe requires the use of both a conventional mortar and pestle, and a Japanese mortar called a suribachi, which has ridges all around the bowl (ideal for grinding seeds, you can find it in Asian food stores and natural food markets). A blender is not a substitute: the grinding has to be done by hand for flavorful results. Sprinkle liberally over cooked grain dishes and vegetables, or use 1 to 2 teaspoons per day as a snack, pick-me-up, or mineral supplement. You can also find already-prepared variations of this recipe in health food stores; just check the macrobiotic foods section.

1   cup sesame seeds with hulls
     small handfuls (about 1/2 ounce) dried wakame seaweed

1. Preheat the oven to 350 degrees F. Wash the sesame seeds and drain thoroughly in a strainer. Toast in a 1-quart metal saucepan, stirring all the time, until they begin to pop energetically and turn aromatic. (Do not wait for the seeds to change color, because they might burn.)
2. Place the wakame seaweed on a cookie sheet, and toast in the oven for about 10 minutes, or until dry and brittle. Remove from the oven and cool. Break gently into a marble or wood mortar. Grind with a pestle until powdery. Discard all unbroken tough stems.
3. Place the sesame seeds into the suribachi and grind for 2 to 3 minutes. Add 2 tablespoons of the wakame powder, and continue grinding for 2 to 3 minutes, or until 70 to 80 percent of the seeds are broken up. Store in an airtight container. Makes about 1 cup.

Toasted Nori

1   sheet nori seaweed

Toast the nori by holding it 3 to 4 inches over a gas flame and turning it until it shrinks and turns dark, 1 to 2 minutes. You can also toast the nori in a toaster oven: fold it over and toast at the lowest setting. Eat as is, cut into strips, or rip into small pieces and sprinkle over grain. Makes 2 servings.

Green Drink

This is my version of the calcium-rich vegetable drink that Nina Merer used daily to strengthen her bones (see chapter 7). Ideally, all vegetables should be organically grown for higher nutrient value and better taste. Here are some optional additions: 1/2 apple, 1 to 2 slices ginger, 1 raw garlic clove. You can keep it in the refrigerator for 3 days.

- 1 carrot, scrubbed and cut up
- 1 small head romaine lettuce, green part only (about 2 cups)
- 2 large bunches of parsley, washed and dried, coarse stems removed (about 4 cups)
- 2 red radishes, cut up
- 1 celery stalk, cut up
- 6 to 8 cups spring water
- 1 cup fresh orange juice (optional)
- 8 teaspoons flaxseed oil

1. Place the vegetables in batches in the blender (do not fill more than half full), with about 1 1/2 cups of water each time, and process until smooth. Add all the batches into one large bowl and mix well with a spoon. Add the orange juice.
2. Just before serving, add 1 teaspoon flaxseed oil to each portion. Drink 1 or 2 cups each day.

Makes about 8 cups

Dr. Corsello's Salad Oil Mix

Serafina Corsello, M.D., recommends this important source of omega-3 fatty acids as the main oil in salad dressings, adding your own favorite herbs.

8   ounces extra virgin olive oil
8   ounces flaxseed oil

Mix the oils in a bottle and keep in the refrigerator. (Also keep the component oils in the refrigerator.)

Other Nutrient Boosters

To add some extra minerals to any dish, use 1 teaspoon to 1 tablespoon per serving of any of the following:

Agar flakes (add to soups before cooking, 1 tablespoon per 4 cups liquid)
Parmesan cheese (before serving)
Chopped fresh parsley (before serving)
Toasted sesame seeds, ground slightly (before serving)
Seaweed sprinkles garnish (available in health food stores)

Menus

When planning a menu, try to include the following:

- a whole grain or whole-grain flour dish
- a source of protein, either beans, fish, chicken, eggs, or meat
- one or more green vegetables
- one or more red or orange vegetables
- a source of good-quality fatty acids

Dessert is optional. Drinks are up to you—just make sure you drink enough water and avoid soft drinks and caffeine. The above guidelines can be combined in just a few dishes if you eat soups or stews.

Here are some suggested combinations of the recipes in this chapter to give you an idea of what I mean. You can look up their nutritional value as complete meals at the end of the nutrition charts section.

Winter Breakfast

Creamy Millet Breakfast Porridge (page 148)

Winter Lunch

Chicken Soup (page 118)
French Tart with Greens and Leeks (page 144)
Cucumber and Radish Salad with Wakame and Walnut-Lime Dressing (page 126)

Winter Dinner

Miso Soup with Wild Mushrooms and Garlic (page 117)
Poached Red Snapper Fillets with Parsley Sauce (page 159)
Puree of Yams (page 142)
Steamed brown rice with Sesame Seaweed Sprinkle (page 170)
Broiled Bananas (page 167)

Meatless Winter Lunch

Root Stew with White Beans and Chanterelles (page 154)
Curried Mustard Greens with Parmesan (page 136)
Plain Kasha (page 149)

Meatless Winter Dinner

Vegetable soup
Flavorful Rice and Barley (page 146)
Anasazi Beans with Collards and Shiitake (page 156)
Steamed carrots
Almond Milk Pudding (page 166)

Summer Breakfast

Fresh Fruit Salad with Toasted Sunflower Seeds (page 129)
Oat-Dulse Crackers (page 153)

Summer Lunch

Salmon Omelet with Fresh Dill (page 161)
Broccoli with Mushrooms (page 139)
Whole-grain toast

Summer Dinner

Cucumber-Avocado Soup (page 115)
Stir-fried Bok Choy with Shrimp (page 134)
Polenta (page 151)
Raw carrot sticks or baby carrots
Apple-strawberry Mold (page 165) with slivered almonds

Meatless Summer Lunch

Chickpea Tabbouleh (page 124)
2 ears corn on the cob with 1 teaspoon organic unsalted butter

Meatless Summer Dinner

Composed Salad with Beets and Avocado (page 127)
Flavorful Rice and Barley (page 146)
Miso-broiled Tofu (page 137)
Asparagus with Slivered Almonds (page 131)
Fresh figs

Chicken Dinner

    Cabbage and Celery Soup (page 116)
    Tossed green salad with olive oil and lemon juice
    Roasted chicken
    Kasha with Mushrooms (page 150)
    Baked Buttercup Squash (page 140)

These are only suggestions, and they may provide too much food for some people, and too little for others. Adjust, mix, and create your own colorful, nutritious meals based on your own tastes and needs.

Appendix: Nutritional Information on Recipes and Menus

In this section, you will find complete nutritional information for each recipe, compared to the needs of a fifty-five-year-old "average woman." The bar graphs and data, except as noted, are from The Food Processor® Nutrition Analysis Software from ESHA Research, Salem, Oregon. Recipes marked by an asterisk (*) were individually analyzed for calcium, magnesium, potassium, sodium, and zinc content by Southern Testing and Research Laboratories in Wilson, North Carolina. Additional nutritional information, mostly regarding the nutrient value of seaweeds, was obtained from *The Nutrition Almanac*, by Lavon J. Dunne. All the stocks were analyzed privately. I then added them to the FP database, so that when I analyzed a soup, for example, I had the additional nutrients from chicken stock.

A word about the reliability of the numbers in nutritional data: *These are figures that correspond to the foods that were analyzed in a laboratory; they do not necessarily correspond to what is found on your dinner plate.* The foods you actually eat may have higher or lower amounts of each nutrient. Therefore, it is impossible to know exactly how much you are getting of any nutrient. While it is interesting and fun to analyze and interpret these numbers—and, believe me, I greatly enjoyed the process of coming up with the bar graphs—they should not be taken as gospel, only as approximations. Counting nutrients exactly to the gram and milligram is not only unrealistic but impossible. Just remember, regardless of the numbers, food is still food, and no matter how the numbers add up it should still be delicious and comforting.

Stocks*

Milligrams (mg) per 100 grams

Type	Calcium	Magnesium	Potassium	Sodium	Zinc
Vegetable	5.33	5.18	112	16.2	0.165
Fish	8.07	4.46	82.6	28.1	0.207
Shrimp	10.4	3.13	51.9	22.8	0.192
Chicken	6.08	1.88	47.7	8.64	0.191
Beef	10.8	3.76		18.2	0.0865

Whenever a recipe calls for a choice of stock or water, the analysis was done with vegetable stock.

Almond Milk Pudding

Serving size: 120.95 g (4.27 oz-wt.)   Serves: 4

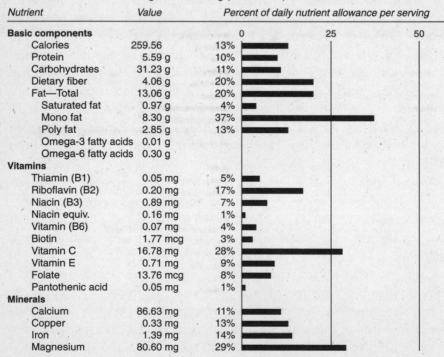

Nutrient	Value	Percent of daily nutrient allowance per serving
Basic components		
Calories	259.56	13%
Protein	5.59 g	10%
Carbohydrates	31.23 g	11%
Dietary fiber	4.06 g	20%
Fat—Total	13.06 g	20%
Saturated fat	0.97 g	4%
Mono fat	8.30 g	37%
Poly fat	2.85 g	13%
Omega-3 fatty acids	0.01 g	
Omega-6 fatty acids	0.30 g	
Vitamins		
Thiamin (B1)	0.05 mg	5%
Riboflavin (B2)	0.20 mg	17%
Niacin (B3)	0.89 mg	7%
Niacin equiv.	0.16 mg	1%
Vitamin (B6)	0.07 mg	4%
Biotin	1.77 mcg	3%
Vitamin C	16.78 mg	28%
Vitamin E	0.71 mg	9%
Folate	13.76 mcg	8%
Pantothenic acid	0.05 mg	1%
Minerals		
Calcium	86.63 mg	11%
Copper	0.33 mg	13%
Iron	1.39 mg	14%
Magnesium	80.60 mg	29%

Almond Milk Pudding *continued*

Nutrient	Value	Percent of daily nutrient allowance per serving		

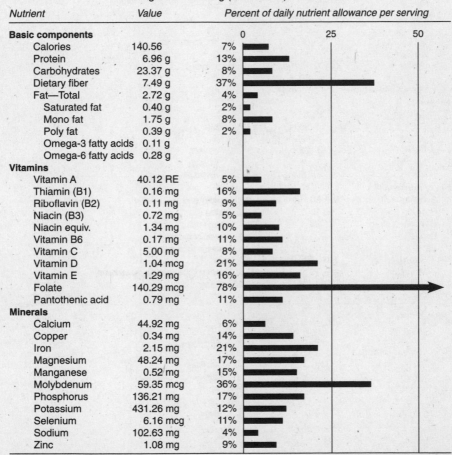

Minerals *continued*

		0	25	50
Manganese	0.44 mg	13%		
Phosphorus	137.06 mg	17%		
Potassium	207.89 mg	6%		
Selenium	0.54 mcg	1%		
Zinc	1.36 mg	11%		

Anasazi Beans with Collards and Shiitake

Serving size: 136.33 g (4.81 oz-wt.)   Serves: 6

Nutrient	Value	Percent of daily nutrient allowance per serving

Basic components

		0	25	50
Calories	140.56	7%		
Protein	6.96 g	13%		
Carbohydrates	23.37 g	8%		
Dietary fiber	7.49 g	37%		
Fat—Total	2.72 g	4%		
Saturated fat	0.40 g	2%		
Mono fat	1.75 g	8%		
Poly fat	0.39 g	2%		
Omega-3 fatty acids	0.11 g			
Omega-6 fatty acids	0.28 g			

Vitamins

Vitamin A	40.12 RE	5%		
Thiamin (B1)	0.16 mg	16%		
Riboflavin (B2)	0.11 mg	9%		
Niacin (B3)	0.72 mg	5%		
Niacin equiv.	1.34 mg	10%		
Vitamin B6	0.17 mg	11%		
Vitamin C	5.00 mg	8%		
Vitamin D	1.04 mcg	21%		
Vitamin E	1.29 mg	16%		
Folate	140.29 mcg	78%		
Pantothenic acid	0.79 mg	11%		

Minerals

Calcium	44.92 mg	6%		
Copper	0.34 mg	14%		
Iron	2.15 mg	21%		
Magnesium	48.24 mg	17%		
Manganese	0.52 mg	15%		
Molybdenum	59.35 mcg	36%		
Phosphorus	136.21 mg	17%		
Potassium	431.26 mg	12%		
Selenium	6.16 mcg	11%		
Sodium	102.63 mg	4%		
Zinc	1.08 mg	9%		

Apple-Strawberry Mold

Serving size: 132.78 g (4.68 oz-wt.)   Serves: 4

Nutrient	Value	Percent of daily nutrient allowance per serving
Basic components		0 25 50
Calories	54.96	3%
Protein	0.27 g	1%
Carbohydrates	13.38 g	5%
Dietary fiber	0.49 g	2%
Poly fat	0.12 g	1%
Omega-3 fatty acids	0.01 g	
Omega-6 fatty acids	0.01 g	
Vitamins		
Thiamin (B1)	0.02 mg	2%
Riboflavin (B2)	0.03 mg	3%
Niacin (B3)	0.18 mg	1%
Vitamin B6	0.04 mg	3%
Vitamin C	9.65 mg	16%
Vitamin E	0.14 mg	2%
Folate	12.66 mcg	7%
Vitamin K	1.68 mcg	2%
Pantothenic acid	0.08 mg	1%
Minerals		
Calcium	19.13 mg	2%
Copper	0.05 mg	2%
Iodine	1.08 mcg	1%
Iron	0.85 mg	8%
Magnesium	19.08 mg	7%
Manganese	0.30 mg	9%
Phosphorus	11.38 mg	1%
Potassium	170.84 mg	5%
Zinc	0.16 mg	1%

Asparagus with Slivered Almonds

Serving Size: 64.33 g (2.27 oz-wt.)   Serves: 4

Nutrient	Value	Percent of daily nutrient allowance per serving
Basic components		0 25 50
Calories	64.63	3%
Protein	3.21 g	6%
Carbohydrates	4.01 g	1%
Dietary fiber	1.68 g	8%
Fat—Total	4.47 g	7%
Saturated fat	0.34 g	2%
Mono fat	2.76 g	12%
Poly fat	1.00 g	5%
Omega-3 fatty acids	0.00 g	
Omega-6 fatty acids	0.07 g	
Vitamins		
Vitamin A	30.18 RE	4%
Thiamin (B1)	0.08 mg	8%
Riboflavin (B2)	0.13 mg	11%
Niacin (B3)	0.87 mg	7%
Niacin equiv.	0.23 mg	2%

Asparagus with Slivered Almonds *continued*

Nutrient	Value	Percent of daily nutrient allowance per serving
		0 25 50
Vitamins *continued*		
Vitamin B6	0.08 mg	5%
Vitamin C	6.04 mg	10%
Vitamin E	0.56 mg	7%
Folate	84.90 mcg	47%
Vitamin K	28.51 mcg	42%
Pantothenic acid	0.09 mg	1%
Minerals		
Calcium	32.44 mg	4%
Copper	0.16 mg	6%
Iron	0.72 mg	7%
Magnesium	31.24 mg	11%
Manganese	0.08 mg	2%
Phosphorus	75.16 mg	9%
Potassium	142.59 mg	4%
Selenium	0.95 mcg	2%
Zinc	0.53 mg	4%

Baked Buttercup Squash

Serving size: 154.60 g (5.45 oz-wt.)   Serves: 4

Nutrient	Value	Percent of daily nutrient allowance per serving
		0 25 50
Basic components		
Calories	102.08	5%
Protein	1.56 g	3%
Carbohydrates	19.99 g	7%
Dietary fiber	6.02 g	30%
Fat—Total	3.07 g	5%
Saturated fat	1.83 g	8%
Mono fat	0.86 g	4%
Poly fat	0.19 g	1%
Omega-3 fatty acids	0.09 g	
Omega-6 fatty acids	0.10 g	
Cholesterol	7.77 mg	3%
Vitamins		
Vitamin A	85.60 RE	11%
Thiamin (B1)	0.23 mg	23%
Riboflavin (B2)	0.02 mg	2%
Niacin (B3)	1.21 mg	9%
Niacin equiv.	0.37 mg	3%
Vitamin B6	0.27 mg	17%
Vitamin C	14.78 mg	25%
Vitamin D	0.05 mcg	1%
Vitamin E	0.96 mg	12%
Folate	25.69 mcg	14%
Pantothenic acid	0.69 mg	10%
Minerals		
Calcium	61.81 mg	8%
Copper	0.12 mg	5%
Iron	1.28 mg	13%
Magnesium	59.66 mg	21%

Baked Buttercup Squash *continued*

Nutrient	Value	Percent of daily nutrient allowance per serving			
		0	25		50
Minerals *continued*					
Manganese	0.33 mg	9%			
Phosphorus	62.40 mg	8%			
Potassium	614.94 mg	16%			
Selenium	1.79 mcg	3%			
Zinc	0.26 mg	2%			

Basic Garlic Greens

Serving size: 97.81 g (3.45 oz-wt.)   Serves: 4

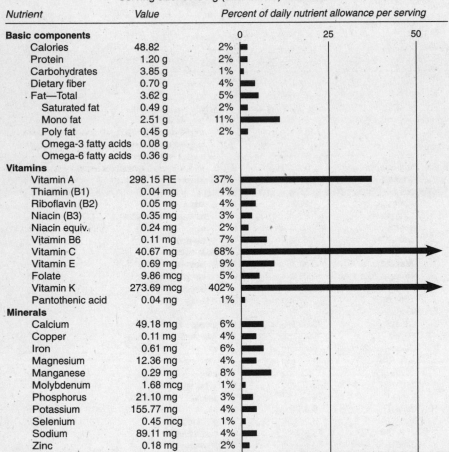

Nutrient	Value	Percent of daily nutrient allowance per serving			
		0	25		50
Basic components					
Calories	48.82	2%			
Protein	1.20 g	2%			
Carbohydrates	3.85 g	1%			
Dietary fiber	0.70 g	4%			
Fat—Total	3.62 g	5%			
Saturated fat	0.49 g	2%			
Mono fat	2.51 g	11%			
Poly fat	0.45 g	2%			
Omega-3 fatty acids	0.08 g				
Omega-6 fatty acids	0.36 g				
Vitamins					
Vitamin A	298.15 RE	37%			
Thiamin (B1)	0.04 mg	4%			
Riboflavin (B2)	0.05 mg	4%			
Niacin (B3)	0.35 mg	3%			
Niacin equiv.	0.24 mg	2%			
Vitamin B6	0.11 mg	7%			
Vitamin C	40.67 mg	68%			
Vitamin E	0.69 mg	9%			
Folate	9.86 mcg	5%			
Vitamin K	273.69 mcg	402%			
Pantothenic acid	0.04 mg	1%			
Minerals					
Calcium	49.18 mg	6%			
Copper	0.11 mg	4%			
Iron	0.61 mg	6%			
Magnesium	12.36 mg	4%			
Manganese	0.29 mg	8%			
Molybdenum	1.68 mcg	1%			
Phosphorus	21.10 mg	3%			
Potassium	155.77 mg	4%			
Selenium	0.45 mcg	1%			
Sodium	89.11 mg	4%			
Zinc	0.18 mg	2%			

Broccoli Rabe with Roasted Garlic plus Red Pepper

Serving size: 108.04 g (3.81 oz-wt.)   Serves: 6

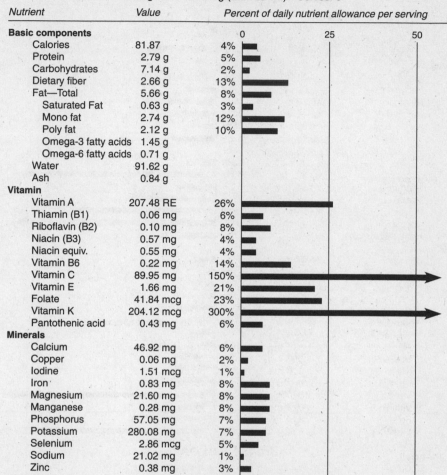

Nutrient	Value	Percent of daily nutrient allowance per serving
Basic components		
Calories	81.87	4%
Protein	2.79 g	5%
Carbohydrates	7.14 g	2%
Dietary fiber	2.66 g	13%
Fat—Total	5.66 g	8%
Saturated Fat	0.63 g	3%
Mono fat	2.74 g	12%
Poly fat	2.12 g	10%
Omega-3 fatty acids	1.45 g	
Omega-6 fatty acids	0.71 g	
Water	91.62 g	
Ash	0.84 g	
Vitamin		
Vitamin A	207.48 RE	26%
Thiamin (B1)	0.06 mg	6%
Riboflavin (B2)	0.10 mg	8%
Niacin (B3)	0.57 mg	4%
Niacin equiv.	0.55 mg	4%
Vitamin B6	0.22 mg	14%
Vitamin C	89.95 mg	150%
Vitamin E	1.66 mg	21%
Folate	41.84 mcg	23%
Vitamin K	204.12 mcg	300%
Pantothenic acid	0.43 mg	6%
Minerals		
Calcium	46.92 mg	6%
Copper	0.06 mg	2%
Iodine	1.51 mcg	1%
Iron	0.83 mg	8%
Magnesium	21.60 mg	8%
Manganese	0.28 mg	8%
Phosphorus	57.05 mg	7%
Potassium	280.08 mg	7%
Selenium	2.86 mcg	5%
Sodium	21.02 mg	1%
Zinc	0.38 mg	3%

Broccoli with Mushrooms

Serving size: 121.60 g (4.29 oz-wt.)   Serves: 4

Nutrient	Value	Percent of daily nutrient allowance per serving
Basic components		
Calories	63.80	3%
Protein	3.31 g	6%
Carbohydrates	6.43 g	2%
Dietary fiber	3.01 g	15%
Fat—Total	3.81 g	6%
Saturated fat	0.52 g	2%
Mono fat	2.51 g	11%

184 Appendix

Broccoli with Mushrooms *continued*

Nutrient	Value	Percent of daily nutrient allowance per serving
Basic Components *continued*		0 / 25 / 50
Poly fat	0.53 g	2%
Omega-3 fatty acids	0.14 g	
Omega-6 fatty acids	0.39 g	
Vitamins		
Vitamin A	135.52 RE	17%
Thiamin (B1)	0.09 mg	9%
Riboflavin (B2)	0.23 mg	19%
Niacin (B3)	1.74 mg	13%
Niacin equiv.	0.66 mg	5%
Vitamin B6	0.19 mg	12%
Vitamin B12	0.00 mcg	0%
Biotin	4.98 mcg	8%
Vitamin C	83.48 mg	139%
Vitamin D	0.54 mcg	11%
Vitamin E	1.97 mg	25%
Folate	68.51 mcg	38%
Vitamin K	180.41 mcg	265%
Pantothenic acid	1.10 mg	16%
Minerals		
Calcium	46.47 mg	6%
Chromium	1.98 mcg	2%
Copper	0.18 mg	7%
Iodine	2.61 mcg	2%
Iron	1.17 mg	12%
Magnesium	25.21 mg	9%
Manganese	0.26 mg	7%
Molybdenum	5.82 mcg	4%
Phosphorus	89.90 mg	11%
Potassium	396.94 mg	11%
Selenium	6.52 mcg	12%
Sodium	170.49 mg	7%
Zinc	0.58 mg	5%

Broiled Bananas

Serving size: 149.22 g (5.26 oz-wt.)   Serves: 2

Nutrient	Value	Percent of daily nutrient allowance per serving
Basic components		0 / 25 / 50
Calories	190.88	10%
Protein	1.23 g	2%
Carbohydrates	34.33 g	12%
Dietary fiber	2.83 g	14%
Fat—Total	6.96 g	10%
Saturated fat	4.20 g	19%
Mono fat	1.89 g	9%
Poly fat	0.35 g	2%
Omega-3 fatty acids	0.13 g	
Omega-6 fatty acids	0.22 g	
Cholesterol	16.40 mg	5%

Broiled Bananas *continued*

Nutrient	Value	Percent of daily nutrient allowance per serving
Vitamins		
Vitamin A	68.70 RE	9%
Thiamin (B1)	0.05 mg	5%
Riboflavin (B2)	0.12 mg	10%
Niacin (B3)	0.64 mg	5%
Niacin equiv.	0.24 mg	2%
Vitamin B6	0.68 mg	43%
Vitamin B12	0.00 mcg	0%
Biotin	3.07 mcg	5%
Vitamin C	10.74 mg	18%
Vitamin D	0.12 mcg	2%
Vitamin E	0.57 mg	7%
Folate	22.55 mcg	13%
Vitamin K	1.18 mcg	2%
Pantothenic acid	0.31 mg	4%
Minerals		
Calcium	14.33 mg	2%
Copper	0.13 mg	5%
Iodine	9.44 mcg	6%
Iron	0.49 mg	5%
Magnesium	35.80 mg	13%
Manganese	0.51 mg	15%
Phosphorus	23.99 mg	3%
Potassium	487.99 mg	13%
Selenium	1.27 mcg	2%
Zinc	0.61 mg	5%

Butternut Squash with Onions and Tarragon

Serving size: 127.98 g (4.51 oz-wt.)   Serves: 5

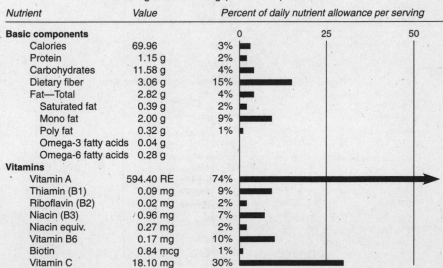

Nutrient	Value	Percent of daily nutrient allowance per serving
Basic components		
Calories	69.96	3%
Protein	1.15 g	2%
Carbohydrates	11.58 g	4%
Dietary fiber	3.06 g	15%
Fat—Total	2.82 g	4%
Saturated fat	0.39 g	2%
Mono fat	2.00 g	9%
Poly fat	0.32 g	1%
Omega-3 fatty acids	0.04 g	
Omega-6 fatty acids	0.28 g	
Vitamins		
Vitamin A	594.40 RE	74%
Thiamin (B1)	0.09 mg	9%
Riboflavin (B2)	0.02 mg	2%
Niacin (B3)	0.96 mg	7%
Niacin equiv.	0.27 mg	2%
Vitamin B6	0.17 mg	10%
Biotin	0.84 mcg	1%
Vitamin C	18.10 mg	30%

Butternut Squash with Onions and Tarragon *continued*

Nutrient	Value	Percent of daily nutrient allowance per serving		
		0	25	50
Vitamins *continued*				
Vitamin E	0.56 mg	7%		
Folate	24.96 mcg	14%		
Vitamin K	0.48 mcg	-1%		
Pantothenic acid	0.34 mg	5%		
Minerals				
Calcium	45.99 mg	6%		
Chromium	3.72 mcg	3%		
Copper	0.07 mg	3%		
Iron	0.63 mg	6%		
Magnesium	29.94 mg	11%		
Manganese	0.22 mg	6%		
Molybdenum	5.01 mcg	3%		
Phosphorus	35.85 mg	4%		
Potassium	338.59 mg	9%		
Selenium	0.62 mcg	1%		
Sodium	240.30 mg	10%		
Zinc	0.22 mg	2%		

Cabbage and Celery Soup

Serving size: 226.94 g (8.01 oz-wt.)   Serves: 8

Nutrient	Value	Percent of daily nutrient allowance per serving		
		0	25	50
Basic components				
Calories	23.33	1%		
Protein	0.62 g	1%		
Carbohydrates	3.59 g	1%		
Dietary fiber	1.26 g	6%		
Fat—Total	0.95 g	1%		
Saturated fat	0.13 g	1%		
Mono fat	0.63 g	3%		
Poly fat	0.13 g	1%		
Omega-3 fatty acids	0.02 g			
Omega-6 fatty acids	0.11 g			
Vitamins				
Vitamin A	257.39 RE	32%		
Thiamin (B1)	0.03 mg	3%		
Riboflavin (B2)	0.02 mg	2%		
Niacin (B3)	0.20 mg	2%		
Niacin equiv.	0.12 mg	1%		
Vitamin B6	0.06 mg	4%		
Biotin	1.30 mcg	2%		
Vitamin C	8.40 mg	14%		
Vitamin E	0.60 mg	8%		
Folate	15.60 mcg	9%		
Vitamin K	13.32 mcg	20%		
Pantothenic acid	0.08 mg	1%		
Minerals				
Calcium	28.65 mg	4%		
Chromium	2.13 mcg	2%		
Copper	0.02 mg	1%		

Cabbage and Celery Soup *continued*

Nutrient	Value	Percent of daily nutrient allowance per serving		
		0	25	50
Minerals *continued*				
Iron	0.24 mg	2%		
Magnesium	15.82 mg	6%		
Manganese	0.08 mg	2%		
Molybdenum	2.76 mcg	2%		
Phosphorus	16.28 mg	2%		
Potassium	327.33 mg	9%		
Selenium	0.57 mcg	1%		
Sodium	338.00 mg	14%		
Zinc	0.38 mg	3%		

Cajun Kale with Carrots and Turnip

Serving size: 247.25 g (8.72 oz-wt.)   Serves: 6

Nutrient	Value	Percent of daily nutrient allowance per serving		
		0	25	50
Basic components				
Calories	80.13	4%		
Protein	2.16 g	4%		
Carbohydrates	13.10 g	5%		
Dietary fiber	3.54 g	18%		
Fat—Total	2.62 g	4%		
Saturated fat	0.36 g	2%		
Mono fat	1.69 g	8%		
Poly fat	0.40 g	2%		
Omega-3 fatty acids	0.09 g			
Omega-6 fatty acids	0.30 g			
Vitamins				
Vitamin A	1623.66 RE	203%		
Thiamin (B1)	0.07 mg	7%		
Riboflavin (B2)	0.08 mg	7%		
Niacin (B3)	0.71 mg	5%		
Niacin equiv.	0.42 mg	3%		
Vitamin B6	0.26 mg	16%		
Biotin	3.58 mcg	6%		
Vitamin C	31.23 mg	52%		
Vitamin E	1.04 mg	13%		
Folate	24.83 mcg	14%		
Vitamin K	9.93 mcg	15%		
Pantothenic acid	0.30 mg	4%		
Minerals				
Calcium	72.37 mg	9%		
Chromium	4.13 mcg	3%		
Copper	0.20 mg	8%		
Iron	0.94 mg	9%		
Magnesium	26.56 mg	9%		
Manganese	0.68 mg	19%		
Molybdenum	3.50 mcg	2%		
Phosphorus	49.26 mg	6%		
Potassium	434.32 mg	12%		
Selenium	0.99 mcg	2%		
Sodium	280.98 mg	12%		
Zinc	0.56 mg	5%		

Chicken Soup

Serving size: 287.68 g (10.15 oz-wt.)   Serves: 4

Nutrient	Value	Percent of daily nutrient allowance per serving
Basic components		
Calories	54.73	3%
Protein	6.73 g	12%
Carbohydrates	3.70 g	1%
Dietary fiber	1.11 g	6%
Fat—Total	1.39 g	2%
Saturated fat	0.36 g	2%
Mono fat	0.46 g	2%
Poly fat	0.34 g	2%
Omega-3 fatty acids	0.03 g	
Omega-6 fatty acids	0.30 g	
Cholesterol	20.24 mg	7%
Vitamins		
Vitamin A	1022.01 RE	128%
Thiamin (B1)	0.05 mg	5%
Riboflavin (B2)	0.07 mg	6%
Niacin (B3)	1.33 mg	10%
Niacin equiv.	1.30 mg	10%
Vitamin B6	0.11 mg	7%
Vitamin B12	0.06 mcg	3%
Biotin	1.80 mcg	3%
Vitamin C	4.47 mg	7%
Vitamin D	0.07 mcg	1%
Vitamin E	0.34 mg	4%
Folate	8.36 mcg	5%
Vitamin K	53.18 mcg	78%
Pantothenic acid	0.30 mg	4%
Minerals		
Calcium	30.15 mg	4%
Copper	0.04 mg	1%
Iron	0.91 mg	9%
Magnesium	17.61 mg	6%
Manganese	0.06 mg	2%
Molybdenum	1.82 mcg	1%
Phosphorus	78.89 mg	10%
Potassium	275.24 mg	7%
Selenium	6.24 mcg	11%
Sodium	390.54 mg	16%
Zinc	1.21 mg	10%

Chickpea Tabbouleh

Serving size: 180.25 g (6.36 oz-wt.)   Serves: 4

Nutrient	Value	Percent of daily nutrient allowance per serving
Basic components		
Calories	294.54	15%
Protein	10.61 g	19%
Carbohydrates	35.41 g	12%
Dietary fiber	9.96 g	50%
Fat—Total	13.52 g	20%

Chickpea Tabbouleh *continued*

Nutrient	Value	Percent of daily nutrient allowance per serving
Basic Components *continued*		0 25 50
Saturated fat	1.41 g	6%
Mono fat	5.60 g	25%
Poly fat	5.64 g	25%
Omega-3 fatty acids	3.08 g	
Omega-6 fatty acids	2.64 g	
Vitamins		
Vitamin A	81.83 RE	10%
Thiamin (B1)	0.27 mg	27%
Riboflavin (B2)	0.13 mg	11%
Niacin (B3)	1.04 mg	8%
Niacin equiv.	1.78 mg	14%
Vitamin B6	0.33 mg	21%
Biotin	1.42 mcg	2%
Vitamin C	27.19 mg	45%
Vitamin E	2.61 mg	33%
Folate	312.83 mcg	174%
Vitamin K	0.80 mcg	1%
Pantothenic acid	0.91 mg	13%
Minerals		
Calcium	87.79 mg	11%
Chromium	6.20 mcg	5%
Copper	0.47 mg	19%
Iodine	0.80 mcg	1%
Iron	4.21 mg	42%
Magnesium	74.43 mg	27%
Manganese	1.18 mg	34%
Molybdenum	2.09 mcg	1%
Phosphorus	206.05 mg	26%
Potassium	655.63 mg	17%
Selenium	4.86 mcg	9%
Sodium	325.66 mg	14%
Zinc	2.07 mg	17%

Cilantro–Egg Drop Soup

Serving size: 310.25 g (10.94 oz-wt.)   Serves: 2

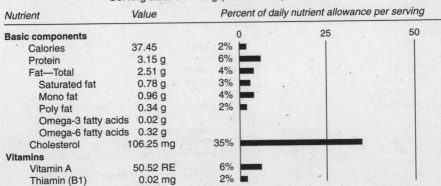

Nutrient	Value	Percent of daily nutrient allowance per serving
Basic components		0 25 50
Calories	37.45	2%
Protein	3.15 g	6%
Fat—Total	2.51 g	4%
Saturated fat	0.78 g	3%
Mono fat	0.96 g	4%
Poly fat	0.34 g	2%
Omega-3 fatty acids	0.02 g	
Omega-6 fatty acids	0.32 g	
Cholesterol	106.25 mg	35%
Vitamins		
Vitamin A	50.52 RE	6%
Thiamin (B1)	0.02 mg	2%

Cilantro–Egg Drop Soup *continued*

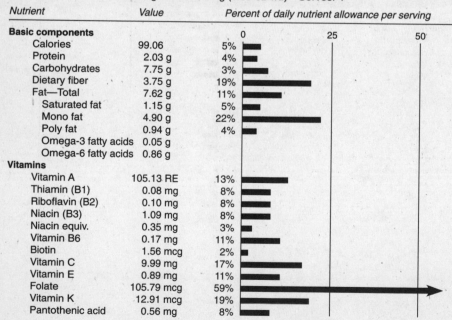

Nutrient	Value	Percent of daily nutrient allowance per serving
Vitamins *continued*		
Riboflavin (B2)	0.13 mg	11%
Niacin equiv.	0.63 mg	5%
Vitamin B6	0.04 mg	2%
Vitamin B12	0.25 mcg	13%
Biotin	5.00 mcg	8%
Vitamin D	0.33 mcg	7%
Vitamin E	0.29 mg	4%
Folate	11.85 mcg	7%
Vitamin K	12.50 mcg	18%
Pantothenic acid	0.32 mg	5%
Minerals		
Calcium	30.65 mg	4%
Iodine	13.25 mcg	9%
Iron	0.38 mg	4%
Magnesium	8.10 mg	3%
Molybdenum	4.25 mcg	3%
Phosphorus	44.86 mg	6%
Potassium	170.96 mg	5%
Selenium	7.72 mcg	14%
Sodium	346.96 mg	14%
Zinc	0.82 mg	7%

Composed Salad with Beets and Avocado

Serving size: 112.60 g (3.97 oz-wt.)   Serves: 4

Nutrient	Value	Percent of daily nutrient allowance per serving
Basic components		
Calories	99.06	5%
Protein	2.03 g	4%
Carbohydrates	7.75 g	3%
Dietary fiber	3.75 g	19%
Fat—Total	7.62 g	11%
Saturated fat	1.15 g	5%
Mono fat	4.90 g	22%
Poly fat	0.94 g	4%
Omega-3 fatty acids	0.05 g	
Omega-6 fatty acids	0.86 g	
Vitamins		
Vitamin A	105.13 RE	13%
Thiamin (B1)	0.08 mg	8%
Riboflavin (B2)	0.10 mg	8%
Niacin (B3)	1.09 mg	8%
Niacin equiv.	0.35 mg	3%
Vitamin B6	0.17 mg	11%
Biotin	1.56 mcg	2%
Vitamin C	9.99 mg	17%
Vitamin E	0.89 mg	11%
Folate	105.79 mcg	59%
Vitamin K	12.91 mcg	19%
Pantothenic acid	0.56 mg	8%

Composed Salad with Beets and Avocado *continued*

Nutrient	Value	Percent of daily nutrient allowance per serving
Minerals		
Calcium	26.85 mg	3%
Copper	0.17 mg	7%
Iodine	0.86 mcg	1%
Iron	1.21 mg	12%
Magnesium	33.97 mg	12%
Manganese	0.40 mg	11%
Phosphorus	44.03 mg	6%
Potassium	497.27 mg	13%
Sodium	44.37 mg	2%
Zinc	0.44 mg	4%

Creamy Lemon-Ginger Dressing

Serving size: 17.83 g (0.63 oz-wt.)   Serves: 16

Nutrient	Value	Percent of daily nutrient allowance per serving		
		0	25	50
Basic components				
Calories	51.37	3%		
Protein	0.59 g	1%		
Dietary fiber	0.12 g	1%		
Fat—Total	5.50 g	8%		
Saturated fat	0.58 g	3%		
Mono fat	2.51 g	11%		
Poly fat	2.32 g	10%		
Omega-3 fatty acids	1.53 g			
Omega-6 fatty acids	0.82 g			
Vitamins				
Thiamin (B1)	0.01 mg	1%		
Niacin equiv.	0.15 mg	1%		
Vitamin C	1.53 mg	3%		
Vitamin E	0.57 mg	7%		
Folate	1.71 mcg	1%		
Minerals				
Calcium	8.02 mg	1%		
Copper	0.02 mg	1%		
Iron	0.40 mg	4%		
Magnesium	7.61 mg	3%		
Manganese	0.04 mg	1%		
Phosphorus	7.39 mg	1%		
Sodium	36.97 mg	2%		
Zinc	0.06 mg	1%		

Creamy Millet Breakfast Porridge

Serving size: 311.19 g (10.98 oz-wt.)   Serves: 4

Nutrient	Value	Percent of daily nutrient allowance per serving
Basic components		
Calories	314.37	16%
Protein	8.69 g	16%
Carbohydrates	40.36 g	14%
Dietary fiber	6.04 g	30%
Fat—Total	13.84 g	21%
Saturated fat	1.43 g	6%
Mono fat	4.65 g	21%
Poly fat	7.10 g	32%
Omega-3 fatty acids	2.09 g	
Omega-6 fatty acids	5.05 g	
Vitamins		
Thiamin (B1)	0.24 mg	24%
Riboflavin (B2)	0.23 mg	19%
Niacin (B3)	3.20 mg	24%
Niacin equiv.	1.76 mg	13%
Vitamin B6	0.27 mg	17%
Biotin	5.21 mcg	8%
Vitamin C	1.91 mg	3%
Vitamin E	6.57 mg	82%
Folate	66.72 mcg	37%
Vitamin K	0.45 mcg	1%
Pantothenic acid	1.03 mg	15%
Minerals		
Calcium	36.40 mg	5%
Copper	0.61 mg	25%
Iodine	1.46 mcg	1%
Iron	2.13 mg	21%
Magnesium	93.98 mg	34%
Manganese	1.17 mg	33%
Molybdenum	2.40 mcg	1%
Phosphorus	277.38 mg	35%
Potassium	229.76 mg	6%
Selenium	6.41 mcg	12%
Sodium	301.47 mg	13%
Zinc	1.57 mg	13%

Crispy Baked Small Fish

Serving size: 85.05 g (3.00 oz-wt.)   Serves: 1

Nutrient	Value	Percent of daily nutrient allowance per serving
Minerals		
Calcium	2829.61 mg	354%
Magnesium	117.37 mg	42%
Potassium	429.50 mg	11%
Sodium	327.44 mg	14%
Zinc	10.29 mg	86%

Crispy Chicken Wings

Serving size: 87.27 g (3.08 oz-wt.)   Serves: 2

Nutrient	Value	Percent of daily nutrient allowance per serving

Basic components

Calories	253.09	13%
Protein	23.48 g	43%
Fat—Total	17.02 g	26%
Saturated fat	4.77 g	21%
Mono fat	6.73 g	30%
Poly fat	3.61 g	16%
Omega-3 fatty acids	0.20 g	
Omega-6 fatty acids	3.25 g	
Cholesterol	73.31 mg	24%

Vitamins

Vitamin A	41.02 RE	5%
Thiamin (B1)	0.04 mg	4%
Riboflavin (B2)	0.11 mg	9%
Niacin (B3)	5.80 mg	44%
Niacin equiv.	4.17 mg	32%
Vitamin B6	0.37 mg	23%
Vitamin B12	0.25 mcg	13%
Vitamin D	0.26 mcg	5%
Vitamin E	1.22 mg	15%
Folate	2.62 mcg	1%
Pantothenic acid	0.78 mg	11%

Minerals

Calcium	13.09 mg	2%
Copper	0.05 mg	2%
Iron	1.11 mg	11%
Magnesium	16.58 mg	6%
Phosphorus	131.78 mg	16%
Potassium	160.58 mg	4%
Selenium	23.21 mcg	42%
Sodium	71.56 mg	3%
Zinc	1.59 mg	13%

Cucumber and Radish Salad with Wakame and Walnut-Lime Dressing

Serving size: 158.00 g (5.57 oz-wt.)   Serves: 4

Nutrient	Value	Percent of daily nutrient allowance per serving

Basic components

Calories	117.12	6%
Protein	1.46 g	3%
Carbohydrates	5.88 g	2%
Dietary fiber	1.14 g	6%
Fat—Total	10.63 g	16%
Saturated fat	0.94 g	4%
Mono fat	2.32 g	10%
Poly fat	6.92 g	31%
Omega-3 fatty acids	2.78 g	
Omega-6 fatty acids	4.20 g	

Vitamins

Vitamin A	31.05 RE	4%
Thiamin (B1)	0.04 mg	4%

Cucumber and Radish Salad with Wakame and Walnut-Lime Dressing *continued*

Nutrient	Value	Percent of daily nutrient allowance per serving
Vitamins *continued*		
Riboflavin (B2)	0.07 mg	6%
Niacin (B3)	0.60 mg	5%
Niacin equiv.	0.21 mg	2%
Vitamin B6	0.06 mg	3%
Biotin	1.02 mcg	2%
Vitamin C	10.37 mg	17%
Vitamin E	2.68 mg	33%
Folate	56.33 mcg	31%
Pantothenic acid	0.36 mg	5%
Minerals		
Calcium	48.00 mg	6%
Copper	0.10 mg	4%
Iron	0.75 mg	8%
Magnesium	34.89 mg	12%
Manganese	0.37 mg	11%
Molybdenum	6.98 mcg	4%
Phosphorus	40.33 mg	5%
Potassium	196.61 mg	5%
Selenium	13.67 mcg	25%
Sodium	323.70 mg	13%
Zinc	0.33 mg	3%

Cucumber-Avocado Soup

Serving size: 291.67 g (10.29 oz-wt.)   Serves: 2

Nutrient	Value	Percent of daily nutrient allowance per serving
Basic components		
Calories	105.99	5%
Protein	3.36 g	6%
Carbohydrates	8.46 g	3%
Dietary fiber	4.06 g	20%
Fat—Total	9.44 g	14%
Saturated fat	1.33 g	6%
Mono fat	5.22 g	23%
Poly fat	0.97 g	4%
Omega-3 fatty acids	0.45 g	
Omega-6 fatty acids	1.83 g	
Vitamins		
Vitamin A	58.04 RE	7%
Thiamin (B1)	0.09 mg	9%
Riboflavin (B2)	0.09 mg	7%
Niacin (B3)	1.19 mg	9%
Niacin equiv.	0.30 mg	2%
Vitamin B6	0.20 mg	13%
Biotin	2.92 mcg	4%
Vitamin C	13.03 mg	22%
Vitamin E	0.96 mg	12%
Folate	48.27 mcg	27%
Vitamin K	11.68 mcg	17%
Pantothenic acid	0.70 mg	10%

Cucumber-Avocado Soup *continued*

Nutrient	Value	Percent of daily nutrient allowance per serving
Minerals		
Calcium	41.00 mg	5%
Copper	0.18 mg	7%
Iodine	0.86 mcg	1%
Iron	1.32 mg	13%
Magnesium	54.70 mg	20%
Manganese	0.25 mg	7%
Molybdenum	7.52 mcg	5%
Phosphorus	85.71 mg	11%
Potassium	537.09 mg	14%
Selenium	20.59 mcg	37%
Zinc	0.81 mg	7%

Curried Mustard Greens with Parmesan

Serving size: 76.87 g (2.71 oz-wt.)   Serves: 4

Nutrient	Value	Percent of daily nutrient allowance per serving
		0 25 50
Basic components		
Calories	95.03	5%
Protein	3.83 g	7%
Carbohydrates	1.97 g	1%
Dietary fiber	0.99 g	5%
Fat—Total	8.37 g	13%
Saturated fat	5.22 g	24%
Mono fat	2.44 g	11%
Poly fat	0.31 g	1%
Omega-3 fatty acids	0.13 g	
Omega-6 fatty acids	0.18 g	
Cholesterol	21.32 mg	7%
Vitamins		
Vitamin A	212.60 RE	27%
Thiamin (B1)	0.03 mg	3%
Riboflavin (B2)	0.06 mg	5%
Niacin (B3)	0.24 mg	2%
Niacin equiv.	0.76 mg	6%
Vitamin B6	0.08 mg	5%
Vitamin B12	0.09 mcg	4%
Vitamin C	12.60 mg	21%
Vitamin D	0.17 mcg	3%
Vitamin E	1.25 mg	16%
Folate	35.11 mcg	20%
Pantothenic acid	0.10 mg	1%
Minerals		
Calcium	126.00 mg	16%
Chloride	115.54 mg	
Copper	0.05 mg	2%
Iron	0.43 mg	4%
Magnesium	11.56 mg	4%
Manganese	0.17 mg	5%
Phosphorus	73.36 mg	9%
Potassium	126.98 mg	3%

Curried Mustard Greens with Parmesan *continued*

Nutrient	Value	Percent of daily nutrient allowance per serving

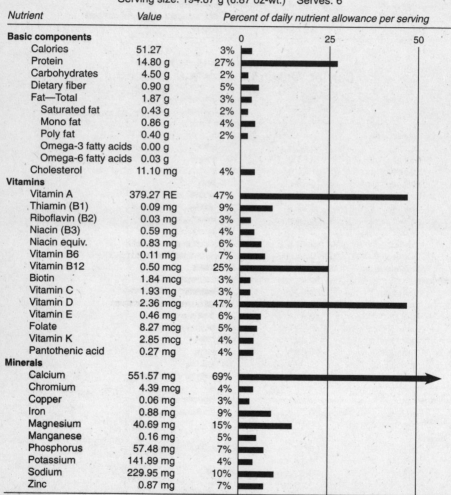

Minerals *continued*

		0	25	50
Selenium	1.63 mcg	3%		
Sodium	417.31 mg	17%		
Zinc	0.30 mg	3%		

5-Hour Whole Fish Soup

Serving size: 194.87 g (6.87 oz-wt.)   Serves: 6

Nutrient	Value	Percent of daily nutrient allowance per serving

Basic components

Nutrient	Value	Percent
Calories	51.27	3%
Protein	14.80 g	27%
Carbohydrates	4.50 g	2%
Dietary fiber	0.90 g	5%
Fat—Total	1.87 g	3%
Saturated fat	0.43 g	2%
Mono fat	0.86 g	4%
Poly fat	0.40 g	2%
Omega-3 fatty acids	0.00 g	
Omega-6 fatty acids	0.03 g	
Cholesterol	11.10 mg	4%

Vitamins

Nutrient	Value	Percent
Vitamin A	379.27 RE	47%
Thiamin (B1)	0.09 mg	9%
Riboflavin (B2)	0.03 mg	3%
Niacin (B3)	0.59 mg	4%
Niacin equiv.	0.83 mg	6%
Vitamin B6	0.11 mg	7%
Vitamin B12	0.50 mcg	25%
Biotin	1.84 mcg	3%
Vitamin C	1.93 mg	3%
Vitamin D	2.36 mcg	47%
Vitamin E	0.46 mg	6%
Folate	8.27 mcg	5%
Vitamin K	2.85 mcg	4%
Pantothenic acid	0.27 mg	4%

Minerals

Nutrient	Value	Percent
Calcium	551.57 mg	69%
Chromium	4.39 mcg	4%
Copper	0.06 mg	3%
Iron	0.88 mg	9%
Magnesium	40.69 mg	15%
Manganese	0.16 mg	5%
Phosphorus	57.48 mg	7%
Potassium	141.89 mg	4%
Sodium	229.95 mg	10%
Zinc	0.87 mg	7%

Appendix

Flavorful Rice and Barley

Serving size: 160.28 g (5.65 oz-wt.)   Serves: 4

Nutrient	Value	Percent of daily nutrient allowance per serving
Basic components		
Calories	166.98	8%
Protein	4.71 g	9%
Carbohydrates	34.76 g	12%
Dietary fiber	4.79 g	24%
Fat—Total	1.20 g	2%
Saturated fat	0.25 g	1%
Mono fat	0.31 g	1%
Poly fat	0.50 g	2%
Omega-3 fatty acids	0.04 g	
Omega-6 fatty acids	0.46 g	
Vitamins		
Thiamin (B1)	0.24 mg	24%
Riboflavin (B2)	0.09 mg	7%
Niacin (B3)	2.24 mg	17%
Niacin equiv.	1.19 mg	9%
Vitamin B6	0.19 mg	12%
Vitamin E	0.61 mg	8%
Folate	9.00 mcg	5%
Vitamin K	0.85 mcg	1%
Pantothenic acid	0.41 mg	6%
Minerals		
Calcium	19.13 mg	2%
Chromium	3.06 mcg	2%
Copper	0.18 mg	7%
Iodine	1.65 mcg	1%
Iron	1.17 mg	12%
Magnesium	69.54 mg	25%
Manganese	1.31 mg	37%
Molybdenum	10.12 mcg	6%
Phosphorus	137.73 mg	17%
Potassium	282.60 mg	8%
Selenium	17.30 mcg	31%
Sodium	313.43 mg	13%
Zinc	1.29 mg	11%

Flax-Apple Shake

Serving size: 733.33 g (25.87 oz-wt.)   Serves: 1

Nutrient	Value	Percent of daily nutrient allowance per serving
Basic components		
Calories	578.82	29%
Protein	7.97 g	15%
Carbohydrates	107.88 g	37%
Dietary fiber	13.78 g	69%
Fat—Total	17.23 g	26%
Saturated fat	1.18 g	8%
Mono fat	0.57 g	3%
Poly fat	2.03 g	9%
Omega-3 fatty acids	1.40 g	
Omega-6 fatty acids	0.67 g	

Flax-Apple Shake *continued*

Nutrient	Value	Percent of daily nutrient allowance per serving
Vitamins		
Vitamin A	12.12 RE	2%
Thiamin (B1)	0.20 mg	20%
Riboflavin (B2)	0.22 mg	18%
Niacin (B3)	1.33 mg	10%
Niacin equiv.	0.25 mg	2%
Vitamin B6	0.56 mg	35%
Biotin	7.23 mcg	11%
Vitamin C	17.70 mg	29%
Vitamin E	1.15 mg	14%
Folate	15.63 mcg	9%
Vitamin K	18.40 mcg	27%
Pantothenic acid	0.55 mg	8%
Minerals		
Calcium	123.92 mg	15%
Copper	0.23 mg	9%
Iodine	4.72 mcg	3%
Iron	4.91 mg	49%
Magnesium	38.89 mg	14%
Manganese	0.71 mg	20%
Phosphorus	56.18 mg	7%
Potassium	1199.72 mg	32%
Selenium	1.80 mcg	3%
Sodium	15.47 mg	1%
Zinc	0.30 mg	2%

French Tart with Greens and Leeks

Serving size: 152.84 g (5.39 oz-wt.)   Serves: 6

Nutrient	Value	Percent of daily nutrient allowance per serving
Basic components		0 25 50
Calories	276.89	14%
Protein	10.86 g	20%
Carbohydrates	25.68 g	9%
Dietary fiber	3.41 g	17%
Fat—Total	15.18 g	23%
Saturated fat	3.90 g	18%
Mono fat	8.64 g	39%
Poly fat	1.67 g	7%
Omega-3 fatty acids	0.19 g	
Omega-6 fatty acids	1.47 g	
Cholesterol	129.81 mg	43%
Vitamins		
Vitamin A	110.27 RE	14%
Thiamin (B1)	0.17 mg	17%
Riboflavin (B2)	0.25 mg	21%
Niacin (B3)	1.85 mg	14%
Niacin equiv.	2.25 mg	17%
Vitamin B6	0.32 mg	20%
Vitamin B12	0.41 mcg	20%
Biotin	7.14 mcg	11%

French Tart with Greens and Leeks *continued*

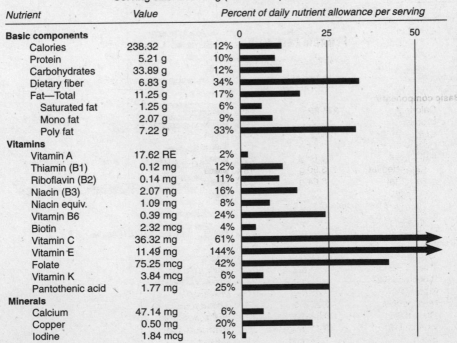

Nutrient	Value	Percent of daily nutrient allowance per serving
Vitamins *continued*		
Vitamin C	25.91 mg	43%
Vitamin D	0.44 mcg	9%
Vitamin E	2.40 mg	30%
Folate	64.07 mcg	36%
Vitamin K	20.85 mcg	31%
Pantothenic acid	0.91 mg	13%
Minerals		
Calcium	172.73 mg	22%
Copper	0.14 mg	6%
Iodine	15.37 mcg	10%
Iron	2.35 mg	23%
Magnesium	54.77 mg	20%
Manganese	1.19 mg	34%
Molybdenum	7.54 mcg	5%
Phosphorus	230.66 mg	29%
Potassium	286.94 mg	8%
Selenium	19.86 mcg	36%
Sodium	403.26 mg	17%
Zinc	1.37 mg	11%

Fresh Fruit Salad with Toasted Sunflower Seeds

Serving size: 219.17 g (7.73 oz-wt.)   Serves: 6

Nutrient	Value	Percent of daily nutrient allowance per serving
Basic components		
Calories	238.32	12%
Protein	5.21 g	10%
Carbohydrates	33.89 g	12%
Dietary fiber	6.83 g	34%
Fat—Total	11.25 g	17%
Saturated fat	1.25 g	6%
Mono fat	2.07 g	9%
Poly fat	7.22 g	33%
Vitamins		
Vitamin A	17.62 RE	2%
Thiamin (B1)	0.12 mg	12%
Riboflavin (B2)	0.14 mg	11%
Niacin (B3)	2.07 mg	16%
Niacin equiv.	1.09 mg	8%
Vitamin B6	0.39 mg	24%
Biotin	2.32 mcg	4%
Vitamin C	36.32 mg	61%
Vitamin E	11.49 mg	144%
Folate	75.25 mcg	42%
Vitamin K	3.84 mcg	6%
Pantothenic acid	1.77 mg	25%
Minerals		
Calcium	47.14 mg	6%
Copper	0.50 mg	20%
Iodine	1.84 mcg	1%

Fresh Fruit Salad with Toasted Sunflower Seeds *continued*

Nutrient	Value	Percent of daily nutrient allowance per serving

Minerals *continued*

Nutrient	Value	Percent
Iron	1.34 mg	13%
Magnesium	46.42 mg	17%
Manganese	0.78 mg	22%
Phosphorus	268.49 mg	34%
Potassium	520.83 mg	14%
Selenium	20.16 mcg	37%
Zinc	1.33 mg	11%

Gingered Kale with Miso-broiled Tofu

Serving size: 113.32 g (4.00 oz-wt.)   Serves: 6

Nutrient	Value	Percent of daily nutrient allowance per serving

Basic components

Nutrient	Value	Percent
Calories	106.61	5%
Protein	10.44 g	19%
Carbohydrates	4.52 g	2%
Dietary fiber	2.45 g	12%
Fat—Total	6.39 g	10%
Saturated fat	0.92 g	4%
Mono fat	2.05 g	9%
Poly fat	3.03 g	14%
Omega-3 fatty acids	0.36 g	
Omega-6 fatty acids	2.67 g	

Vitamins

Nutrient	Value	Percent
Vitamin A	154.23 RE	19%
Thiamin (B1)	0.11 mg	11%
Riboflavin (B2)	0.10 mg	8%
Niacin (B3)	0.45 mg	3%
Niacin equiv.	2.59 mg	20%
Vitamin B6	0.11 mg	7%
Vitamin C	12.62 mg	21%
Vitamin E	1.20 mg	15%
Folate	52.77 mcg	29%
Pantothenic acid	0.14 mg	2%

Minerals

Nutrient	Value	Percent
Calcium	154.07 mg	19%
Copper	0.27 mg	11%
Iron	6.39 mg	64%
Magnesium	62.47 mg	22%
Manganese	0.83 mg	24%
Phosphorus	132.36 mg	17%
Potassium	242.09 mg	6%
Selenium	0.48 mcg	1%
Sodium	125.71 mg	5%
Zinc	1.05 mg	9%

Gingered Vegetable Caviar with Tofu and Dried Mushrooms

Serving size: 146.14 g (5.15 oz-wt.)   Serves: 6

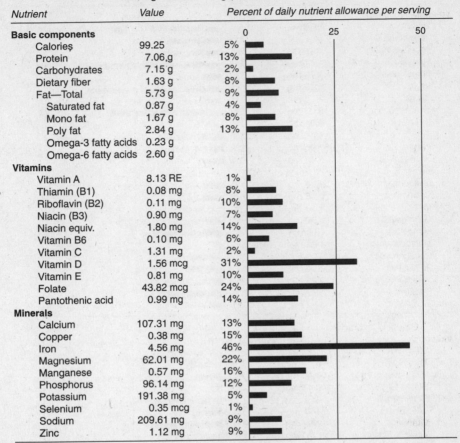

Nutrient	Value	Percent of daily nutrient allowance per serving
Basic components		
Calories	99.25	5%
Protein	7.06 g	13%
Carbohydrates	7.15 g	2%
Dietary fiber	1.63 g	8%
Fat—Total	5.73 g	9%
Saturated fat	0.87 g	4%
Mono fat	1.67 g	8%
Poly fat	2.84 g	13%
Omega-3 fatty acids	0.23 g	
Omega-6 fatty acids	2.60 g	
Vitamins		
Vitamin A	8.13 RE	1%
Thiamin (B1)	0.08 mg	8%
Riboflavin (B2)	0.11 mg	10%
Niacin (B3)	0.90 mg	7%
Niacin equiv.	1.80 mg	14%
Vitamin B6	0.10 mg	6%
Vitamin C	1.31 mg	2%
Vitamin D	1.56 mcg	31%
Vitamin E	0.81 mg	10%
Folate	43.82 mcg	24%
Pantothenic acid	0.99 mg	14%
Minerals		
Calcium	107.31 mg	13%
Copper	0.38 mg	15%
Iron	4.56 mg	46%
Magnesium	62.01 mg	22%
Manganese	0.57 mg	16%
Phosphorus	96.14 mg	12%
Potassium	191.38 mg	5%
Selenium	0.35 mcg	1%
Sodium	209.61 mg	9%
Zinc	1.12 mg	9%

Gratin of Root Vegetables

Serving size: 149.90 g (5.29 oz-wt.)   Serves: 6

Nutrient	Value	Percent of daily nutrient allowance per serving
Basic components		
Calories	145.41	7%
Protein	3.39 g	6%
Carbohydrates	22.28 g	8%
Dietary fiber	3.84 g	19%
Fat—Total	5.51 g	8%
Saturated fat	0.82 g	4%
Mono fat	3.67 g	17%
Poly fat	0.72 g	3%
Omega-3 fatty acids	0.07 g	
Omega-6 fatty acids	0.64 g	

Gratin of Root Vegetables *continued*

Nutrient	Value	Percent of daily nutrient allowance per serving
Vitamins		
Vitamin A	438.88 RE	55%
Thiamin (B1)	0.15 mg	15%
Riboflavin (B2)	0.10 mg	8%
Niacin (B3)	1.47 mg	11%
Niacin equiv.	0.75 mg	6%
Vitamin B6	0.16 mg	10%
Biotin	2.10 mcg	3%
Vitamin C	19.27 mg	32%
Vitamin D	0.04 mcg	1%
Vitamin E	1.06 mg	13%
Folate	31.90 mcg	18%
Pantothenic acid	0.43 mg	6%
Minerals		
Calcium	52.74 mg	7%
Copper	0.15 mg	6%
Iron	1.19 mg	12%
Magnesium	40.56 mg	14%
Manganese	0.81 mg	23%
Molybdenum	1.64 mcg	1%
Phosphorus	100.46 mg	13%
Potassium	380.09 mg	10%
Selenium	9.25 mcg	17%
Sodium	425.87 mg	18%
Zinc	0.82 mg	7%

Green Drink

Serving size: 239.43 g (8.45 oz-wt.)   Serves: 10

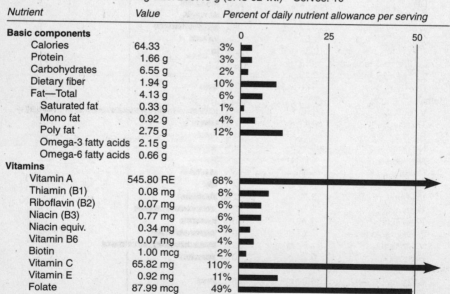

Nutrient	Value	Percent of daily nutrient allowance per serving
		0 25 50
Basic components		
Calories	64.33	3%
Protein	1.66 g	3%
Carbohydrates	6.55 g	2%
Dietary fiber	1.94 g	10%
Fat—Total	4.13 g	6%
Saturated fat	0.33 g	1%
Mono fat	0.92 g	4%
Poly fat	2.75 g	12%
Omega-3 fatty acids	2.15 g	
Omega-6 fatty acids	0.66 g	
Vitamins		
Vitamin A	545.80 RE	68%
Thiamin (B1)	0.08 mg	8%
Riboflavin (B2)	0.07 mg	6%
Niacin (B3)	0.77 mg	6%
Niacin equiv.	0.34 mg	3%
Vitamin B6	0.07 mg	4%
Biotin	1.00 mcg	2%
Vitamin C	65.82 mg	110%
Vitamin E	0.92 mg	11%
Folate	87.99 mcg	49%

Green Drink *continued*

Nutrient	Value	Percent of daily nutrient allowance per serving
Vitamins *continued*		
Vitamin K	16.23 mcg	24%
Pantothenic acid	0.25 mg	4%
Minerals		
Calcium	66.06 mg	8%
Chromium	2.35 mcg	2%
Copper	0.09 mg	3%
Iodine	1.06 mcg	1%
Iron	2.55 mg	26%
Magnesium	25.33 mg	9%
Manganese	0.19 mg	5%
Molybdenum	1.80 mcg	1%
Phosphorus	38.66 mg	5%
Potassium	346.86 mg	9%
Selenium	0.45 mcg	1%
Sodium	33.56 mg	1%
Zinc	0.51 mg	4%

Gumbo

Serving size: 197.67 g (6.97 oz-wt.)   Serves: 6

Nutrient	Value	Percent of daily nutrient allowance per serving
Basic components		
Calories	113.25	6%
Protein	1.84 g	3%
Carbohydrates	13.10 g	5%
Dietary fiber	2.26 g	11%
Fat—Total	6.65 g	10%
Saturated fat	4.03 g	18%
Mono fat	1.87 g	8%
Poly fat	0.36 g	2%
Omega-3 fatty acids	0.13 g	
Omega-6 fatty acids	0.23 g	
Cholesterol	16.40 mg	5%
Vitamins		
Vitamin A	400.65 RE	50%
Thiamin (B1)	0.07 mg	7%
Riboflavin (B2)	0.07 mg	6%
Niacin (B3)	0.96 mg	7%
Niacin equiv.	0.35 mg	3%
Vitamin B6	0.17 mg	10%
Biotin	1.88 mcg	3%
Vitamin C	6.72 mg	11%
Vitamin D	1.16 mcg	23%
Vitamin E	0.76 mg	10%
Folate	32.37 mcg	18%
Vitamin K	21.98 mcg	32%
Pantothenic acid	0.70 mg	10%
Minerals		
Calcium	36.74 mg	5%
Chromium	2.84 mcg	2%

Gumbo *continued*

Nutrient	Value	Percent of daily nutrient allowance per serving

Vitamins *continued*

Nutrient	Value	%
Copper	0.21 mg	8%
Iron	1.01 mg	10%
Magnesium	24.98 mg	9%
Manganese	0.43 mg	12%
Molybdenum	3.33 mcg	2%
Phosphorus	49.75 mg	6%
Potassium	239.14 mg	6%
Selenium	6.21 mcg	11%
Sodium	412.63 mg	17%
Zinc	0.61 mg	5%

Hearty Shrimp Bisque

Serving size: 238.15 g (8.40 oz-wt.)   Serves: 4

Nutrient	Value	Percent of daily nutrient allowance per serving

Basic components

Nutrient	Value	%
Calories	191.42	10%
Protein	10.00 g	18%
Carbohydrates	8.78 g	3%
Dietary fiber	1.62 g	8%
Fat—Total	11.05 g	17%
Saturated fat	1.56 g	7%
Mono fat	7.65 g	34%
Poly fat	1.51 g	7%
Omega-3 fatty acids	0.36 g	
Omega-6 fatty acids	1.06 g	
Cholesterol	63.84 mg	21%

Vitamins

Nutrient	Value	%
Vitamin A	219.22 RE	27%
Thiamin (B1)	0.07 mg	7%
Riboflavin (B2)	0.04 mg	4%
Niacin (B3)	1.69 mg	13%
Niacin equiv.	2.33 mg	18%
Vitamin B6	0.11 mg	7%
Vitamin B12	0.49 mcg	24%
Biotin	1.38 mcg	2%
Vitamin C	3.57 mg	6%
Vitamin D	1.60 mcg	32%
Vitamin E	1.95 mg	24%
Folate	12.01 mcg	7%
Vitamin K	11.42 mcg	17%
Pantothenic acid	0.25 mg	4%

Minerals

Nutrient	Value	%
Calcium	48.35 mg	6%
Chromium	3.10 mcg	2%
Copper	0.16 mg	7%
Iron	1.55 mg	16%
Magnesium	36.46 mg	13%
Manganese	0.49 mg	14%
Molybdenum	1.74 mcg	1%

Hearty Shrimp Bisque *continued*

Nutrient	Value	Percent of daily nutrient allowance per serving

		0	25	50
Minerals *continued*				
Phosphorus	128.09 mg	16%		
Potassium	267.20 mg	7%		
Selenium	21.66 mcg	39%		
Sodium	390.10 mg	16%		
Zinc	1.00 mg	8%		

Kasha with Mushrooms

Serving size: 173.29 g (6.11 oz-wt.)   Serves: 4

Nutrient	Value	Percent of daily nutrient allowance per serving

		0	25	50
Basic components				
Calories	202.82	10%		
Protein	7.54 g	14%		
Carbohydrates	34.99 g	12%		
Dietary fiber	5.55 g	28%		
Fat—Total	5.46 g	8%		
Saturated fat	0.74 g	3%		
Mono fat	1.21 g	5%		
Poly fat	3.08 g	14%		
Omega-3 fatty acids	0.04 g			
Omega-6 fatty acids	3.04 g			
Vitamins				
Thiamin (B1)	0.06 mg	6%		
Riboflavin (B2)	0.25 mg	20%		
Niacin (B3)	4.05 mg	31%		
Niacin equiv.	1.74 mg	13%		
Vitamin B6	0.19 mg	12%		
Vitamin D	1.47 mcg	29%		
Vitamin E	4.47 mg	56%		
Folate	37.49 mcg	21%		
Pantothenic acid	1.86 mg	27%		
Minerals				
Calcium	16.19 mg	2%		
Copper	0.80 mg	32%		
Iron	1.31 mg	13%		
Magnesium	114.37 mg	41%		
Manganese	0.77 mg	22%		
Phosphorus	250.29 mg	31%		
Potassium	317.92 mg	8%		
Selenium	6.28 mcg	11%		
Sodium	295.37 mg	12%		
Zinc	1.75 mg	15%		

Maple-Walnut Loaf

Serving size: 58.81 g (2.07 oz-wt.)   Serves: 12

Nutrient	Value	Percent of daily nutrient allowance per serving
Basic components		
Calories	167.69	8%
Protein	5.75 g	11%
Carbohydrates	18.98 g	7%
Dietary fiber	1.00 g	5%
Fat—Total	8.20 g	12%
Saturated fat	1.10 g	5%
Mono fat	2.17 g	10%
Poly fat	4.28 g	19%
Omega-3 fatty acids	0.37 g	
Omega-6 fatty acids	3.84 g	
Cholesterol	88.54 mg	30%
Vitamins		
Vitamin A	42.80 RE	5%
Thiamin (B1)	0.05 mg	5%
Riboflavin (B2)	0.14 mg	11%
Niacin (B3)	0.37 mg	3%
Niacin equiv.	1.22 mg	9%
Vitamin B6	0.10 mg	6%
Vitamin B12	0.21 mcg	10%
Biotin	6.57 mcg	10%
Vitamin C	0.64 mg	1%
Vitamin D	0.28 mcg	6%
Vitamin E	0.59 mg	7%
Folate	18.89 mcg	10%
Vitamin K	10.42 mcg	15%
Pantothenic acid	0.36 mg	5%
Minerals		
Calcium	32.34 mg	4%
Copper	0.14 mg	6%
Iodine	11.04 mcg	7%
Iron	1.09 mg	11%
Magnesium	31.44 mg	11%
Manganese	1.24 mg	35%
Molybdenum	6.49 mcg	4%
Phosphorus	98.31 mg	12%
Potassium	144.03 mg	4%
Selenium	11.24 mcg	20%
Sodium	54.90 mg	2%
Zinc	1.52 mg	13%

Miso-broiled Tofu

Serving size: 95.91 g (3.38 oz-wt.)   Serves: 4

Nutrient	Value	Percent of daily nutrient allowance per serving
Basic components		
Calories	146.36	7%
Protein	13.83 g	25%
Carbohydrates	4.82 g	2%
Dietary fiber	2.03 g	10%

Miso-broiled Tofu *continued*

Nutrient	Value	Percent of daily nutrient allowance per serving
Basic components *continued*		0 25 50
Fat—Total	9.31 g	14%
Saturated fat	1.33 g	6%
Mono fat	2.92 g	13%
Poly fat	4.38 g	20%
Omega-3 fatty acids	0.51 g	
Omega-6 fatty acids	3.85 g	
Vitamins		
Vitamin A	14.48 RE	2%
Thiamin (B1)	0.14 mg	14%
Riboflavin (B2)	0.09 mg	8%
Niacin (B3)	0.39 mg	3%
Niacin equiv.	3.49 mg	26%
Vitamin B6	0.08 mg	5%
Vitamin C	0.76 mg	1%
Vitamin E	0.23 mg	3%
Folate	25.08 mcg	14%
Pantothenic acid	0.11 mg	2%
Minerals		
Calcium	178.24 mg	22%
Copper	0.32 mg	13%
Iron	9.06 mg	91%
Magnesium	80.06 mg	29%
Manganese	1.00 mg	29%
Phosphorus	167.37 mg	21%
Potassium	216.35 mg	6%
Sodium	176.65 mg	7%
Zinc	1.35 mg	11%

Miso Soup with Wild Mushrooms and Garlic

Serving size: 146.90 g (5.18 oz-wt.)   Serves: 4

Nutrient	Value	Percent of daily nutrient allowance per serving
Basic components		0 25 50
Calories	81.66	4%
Protein	5.70 g	10%
Carbohydrates	11.38 g	4%
Dietary fiber	1.89 g	9%
Fat—Total	2.08 g	3%
Saturated fat	0.41 g	2%
Mono fat	0.53 g	2%
Poly fat	0.77 g	3%
Omega-3 fatty acids	0.18 g	
Omega-6 fatty acids	0.56 g	
Vitamins		
Thiamin (B1)	0.08 mg	8%
Riboflavin (B2)	0.23 mg	19%
Niacin (B3)	2.57 mg	19%
Niacin equiv.	0.49 mg	4%
Vitamin B6	0.19 mg	12%
Vitamin B12	0.80 mcg	40%

Miso Soup with Wild Mushrooms and Garlic *continued*

Nutrient	Value	Percent of daily nutrient allowance per serving
Vitamins *continued*		
Vitamin C	1.89 mg	3%
Vitamin D mcg	2.94 mcg	59%
Vitamin E	1.52 mg	19%
Folate	42.62 mcg	24%
Vitamin K	6.47 mcg	10%
Pantothenic acid	2.00 mg	29%
Minerals		
Calcium	23.30 mg	3%
Copper	0.52 mg	21%
Iron	0.70 mg	7%
Magnesium	26.10 mg	9%
Manganese	0.35 mg	10%
Phosphorus	118.12 mg	15%
Potassium	325.32 mg	9%
Selenium	1.01 mcg	2%
Sodium	810.50 mg	34%
Zinc	1.23 mg	10%

Mixed Green Salad

Serving size: 79.03 g (2.79 oz-wt.)   Serves: 4

Nutrient	Value	Percent of daily nutrient allowance per serving
Basic components		
Calories	72.39	4%
Protein	1.02 g	2%
Carbohydrates	2.49 g	1%
Dietary fiber	1.36 g	7%
Fat—Total	6.91 g	10%
Saturated fat	0.81 g	4%
Mono fat	3.08 mg	14%
Poly fat	2.74 g	12%
Vitamins		
Vitamin A	150.07 RE	19%
Thiamin (B1)	0.05 mg	5%
Riboflavin (B2)	0.06 mg	5%
Niacin (B3)	0.27 mg	2%
Niacin equiv.	0.15 mg	1%
Vitamin B6	0.05 mg	3%
Vitamin C	10.98 mg	18%
Vitamin E	0.80 mg	10%
Folate	68.97 mcg	38%
Pantothenic acid	0.17 mg	2%
Minerals		
Calcium	32.98 mg	4%
Copper	0.05 mg	2%
Iron	0.77 mg	8%
Magnesium	14.76 mg	5%
Manganese	0.33 mg	9%
Phosphorus	22.08 mg	3%

Mixed Green Salad *continued*

Nutrient	Value	Percent of daily nutrient allowance per serving

Minerals *continued*

		0	25	50
Potassium	206.94 mg	6%		
Sodium	86.95 mg	4%		
Zinc	0.25 mg	2%		

Oat-Dulse Crackers

Serving size: 119.70 g (4.22 oz-wt.)   Serves: 8

Nutrient	Value	Percent of daily nutrient allowance per serving

Basic components

		0	25	50
Calories	266.82	13%		
Protein	8.45 g	16%		
Carbohydrates	22.40 g	8%		
Dietary fiber	5.20 g	26%		
Fat—Total	18.31 g	27%		
Saturated fat	5.49 g	25%		
Mono fat	4.16 g	19%		
Poly fat	6.67 g	30%		
Omega-3 fatty acids	0.14 g			
Omega-6 fatty acids	6.52 g			
Cholesterol	18.64 mg	6%		

Vitamins

		0	25	50
Vitamin A	67.11 RE	8%		
Thiamin (B1)	0.59 mg	59%		
Riboflavin (B2)	0.09 mg	8%		
Niacin (B3)	1.45 mg	11%		
Niacin equiv.	1.98 mg	15%		
Vitamin B6	0.19 mg	12%		
Vitamin B12	0.01 mcg	1%		
Biotin	4.58 mcg	7%		
Vitamin D	0.12 mcg	2%		
Vitamin E	9.50 mg	119%		
Folate	50.88 mcg	28%		
Vitamin K	101.94 mcg	150%		
Pantothenic acid	1.55 mg	22%		

Minerals

		0	25	50
Calcium	237.57 mg	30%		
Copper	0.42 mg	17%		
Iodine	0.79 mcg	1%		
Iron	4.61 mg	46%		
Magnesium	104.51 mg	37%		
Manganese	1.38 mg	40%		
Phosphorus	258.57 mg	32%		
Potassium	227.51 mg	6%		
Selenium	22.97 mcg	42%		
Sodium	148.89 mg	6%		
Zinc	1.77 mg	15%		

Parsley Sauce

Serving size: 48.17 g (1.70 oz-wt.)   Serves: 6

Nutrient	Value	Percent of daily nutrient allowance per serving
Basic components		0 25 50
Calories	50.79	3%
Protein	0.57 g	1%
Carbohydrates	2.87 g	1%
Dietary fiber	0.50 g	3%
Fat—Total	4.33 g	6%
Saturated fat	2.67 g	12%
Mono fat	1.24 g	6%
Poly fat	0.19 g	1%
Omega-3 fatty acids	0.06 g	
Omega-6 fatty acids	0.13 g	
Cholesterol	10.93 mg	4%
Vitamins		
Vitamin A	46.02 RE	6%
Thiamin (B1)	0.02 mg	2%
Riboflavin (B2)	0.01 mg	1%
Niacin (B3)	0.26 mg	2%
Niacin equiv.	0.14 mg	1%
Vitamin B6	0.01 mg	1%
Vitamin C	2.05 mg	3%
Vitamin D	0.08 mcg	2%
Vitamin E	0.24 mg	3%
Folate	3.67 mcg	2%
Pantothenic acid	0.04 mg	1%
Minerals		
Calcium	6.34 mg	1%
Copper	0.02 mg	1%
Iron	0.22 mg	2%
Magnesium	7.56 mg	3%
Manganese	0.14 mg	4%
Phosphorus	13.88 mg	2%
Potassium	54.62 mg	1%
Selenium	2.73 mcg	5%
Sodium	108.48 mg	5%
Zinc	0.20 mg	2%

Pinto Bean Soup with Dill

Serving size: 318.66 g (11.24 oz-wt.)   Serves: 6

Nutrient	Value	Percent of daily nutrient allowance per serving
Basic components		0 25 50
Calories	158.64	8%
Protein	7.42 g	14%
Carbohydrates	27.13 g	9%
Dietary fiber	8.52 g	43%
Fat—Total	2.91 g	4%
Saturated fat	0.43 g	2%
Mono fat	1.82 g	8%
Poly fat	0.44 g	2%

Pinto Bean Soup with Dill *continued*

Nutrient	Value	Percent of daily nutrient allowance per serving
		0 25 50
Basic components *continued*		
Omega-3 fatty acids	0.10 g	
Omega-6 fatty acids	0.34 g	
Vitamins		
Vitamin A	340.74 RE	43%
Thiamin (B1)	0.19 mg	19%
Riboflavin (B2)	0.10 mg	8%
Niacin (B3)	0.60 mg	5%
Niacin equiv.	1.48 mg	11%
Vitamin B6	0.23 mg	14%
Biotin	2.49 mcg	4%
Vitamin C	7.70 mg	13%
Vitamin E	1.41 mg	18%
Folate	153.03 mcg	85%
Vitamin K	18.47 mcg	27%
Pantothenic acid	0.34 mg	5%
Minerals		
Calcium	72.95 mg	9%
Chromium	8.27 mcg	7%
Copper	0.25 mg	10%
Iodine	1.07 mcg	1%
Iron	2.70 mg	27%
Magnesium	57.77 mg	21%
Manganese	0.59 mg	17%
Molybdenum	63.06 mcg	39%
Phosphorus	155.96 mg	19%
Potassium	635.99 mg	17%
Selenium	6.20 mcg	11%
Sodium	38.61 mg	2%
Zinc	1.32 mg	11%

Plain Kasha

Serving size: 123.08 g (4.34 oz-wt.)   Serves: 6

Nutrient	Value	Percent of daily nutrient allowance per serving
		0 25 50
Basic components		
Calories	97.18	5%
Protein	3.77 g	7%
Carbohydrates	20.26 g	7%
Dietary fiber	2.83 g	14%
Fat—Total	0.96 g	1%
Saturated fat	0.21 g	1%
Mono fat	0.29 g	1%
Poly fat	0.29 g	1%
Omega-3 fatty acids	0.02 g	
Omega-6 fatty acids	0.27 g	
Vitamins		
Thiamin (B1)	0.03 mg	3%
Riboflavin (B2)	0.12 mg	10%
Niacin (B3)	1.99 mg	15%
Niacin equiv.	0.91 mg	7%

Plain Kasha *continued*

Nutrient	Value	Percent of daily nutrient allowance per serving

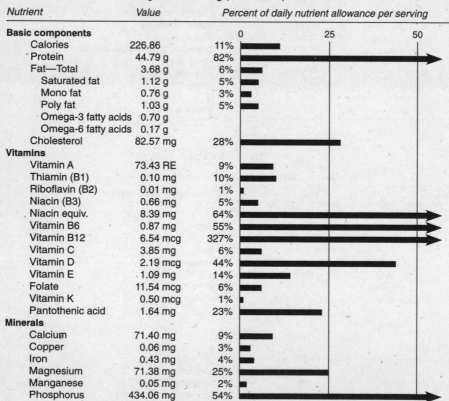

Vitamins *continued*

		0	25	50
Vitamin B6	0.06 mg	4%		
Vitamin E	0.29 mg	4%		
Folate	8.50 mcg	5%		
Pantothenic acid	0.35 mg	5%		

Minerals

Calcium	10.20 mg	1%		
Copper	0.31 mg	12%		
Iron	0.62 mg	6%		
Magnesium	70.35 mg	25%		
Manganese	0.37 mg	11%		
Phosphorus	98.32 mg	12%		
Potassium	236.19 mg	6%		
Sodium	112.49 mg	5%		
Zinc	0.84 mg	7%		

Poached Red Snapper Fillets with Parsley Sauce

Serving size: 233.00 g (8.22 oz-wt.)   Serves: 2

Nutrient	Value	Percent of daily nutrient allowance per serving

Basic components

		0	25	50
Calories	226.86	11%		
Protein	44.79 g	82%		
Fat—Total	3.68 g	6%		
Saturated fat	1.12 g	5%		
Mono fat	0.76 g	3%		
Poly fat	1.03 g	5%		
Omega-3 fatty acids	0.70 g			
Omega-6 fatty acids	0.17 g			
Cholesterol	82.57 mg	28%		

Vitamins

Vitamin A	73.43 RE	9%		
Thiamin (B1)	0.10 mg	10%		
Riboflavin (B2)	0.01 mg	1%		
Niacin (B3)	0.66 mg	5%		
Niacin equiv.	8.39 mg	64%		
Vitamin B6	0.87 mg	55%		
Vitamin B12	6.54 mcg	327%		
Vitamin C	3.85 mg	6%		
Vitamin D	2.19 mcg	44%		
Vitamin E	1.09 mg	14%		
Folate	11.54 mcg	6%		
Vitamin K	0.50 mcg	1%		
Pantothenic acid	1.64 mg	23%		

Minerals

Calcium	71.40 mg	9%		
Copper	0.06 mg	3%		
Iron	0.43 mg	4%		
Magnesium	71.38 mg	25%		
Manganese	0.05 mg	2%		
Phosphorus	434.06 mg	54%		

Poached Red Snapper Fillets with Parsley Sauce *continued*

Nutrient	Value	Percent of daily nutrient allowance per serving
Minerals *continued*		0 25 50
Potassium	924.04 mg	25%
Selenium	83.75 mcg	152%
Sodium	158.89 mg	7%
Zinc	0.83 mg	7%

Polenta

Serving size: 544.03 g (19.19 oz-wt.)   Serves: 2

Nutrient	Value	Percent of daily nutrient allowance per serving
Basic components		0 25 50
Calories	179.17	9%
Protein	3.70 g	7%
Carbohydrates	33.31 g	11%
Dietary fiber	0.51 g	3%
Fat—Total	3.39 g	5%
Saturated fat	1.87 g	8%
Mono fat	0.98 g	4%
Poly fat	0.31 g	1%
Omega-3 fatty acids	0.04 g	
Omega-6 fatty acids	0.27 g	
Cholesterol	7.77 mg	3%
Vitamins		
Vitamin A	42.12 RE	5%
Thiamin (B1)	0.05 mg	5%
Riboflavin (B2)	0.03 mg	2%
Niacin (B3)	0.51 mg	4%
Niacin equiv.	0.43 mg	3%
Vitamin B6	0.06 mg	4%
Vitamin D	0.05 mcg	1%
Vitamin E	0.18 mg	2%
Folate	2.66 mcg	1%
Pantothenic acid	0.17 mg	2%
Minerals		
Calcium	16.12 mg	2%
Copper	0.03 mg	1%
Iron	0.52 mg	5%
Magnesium	25.01 mg	9%
Manganese	0.04 mg	1%
Phosphorus	31.56 mg	4%
Potassium	374.87 mg	10%
Selenium	7.99 mcg	15%
Sodium	337.00 mg	14%
Zinc	0.65 mg	5%

Puree of Yams

Serving size: 130.68 g (4.61 oz-wt.)   Serves: 6

Nutrient	Value	Percent of daily nutrient allowance per serving
Basic components		0 25 50
Calories	123.00	6%
Protein	1.72 g	3%
Carbohydrates	24.30 g	8%
Dietary fiber	2.70 g	14%
Fat—Total	2.44 g	4%
Saturated fat	0.19 g	1%
Mono fat	0.50 g	2%
Poly fat	1.72 g	8%
Omega-3 fatty acids	1.34 g	
Omega-6 fatty acids	0.41 g	
Vitamins		
Vitamin A	2182.00 RE	273%
Thiamin (B1)	0.07 mg	7%
Riboflavin (B2)	0.13 mg	11%
Niacin (B3)	0.60 mg	5%
Niacin equiv.	0.35 mg	3%
Vitamin B6	0.24 mg	15%
Biotin	4.30 mcg	7%
Vitamin C	24.60 mg	41%
Vitamin E	0.28 mg	4%
Folate	22.60 mcg	13%
Pantothenic acid	0.65 mg	9%
Minerals		
Calcium	29.51 mg	4%
Copper	0.21 mg	8%
Iodine	3.00 mcg	2%
Iron	0.45 mg	5%
Magnesium	21.47 mg	8%
Manganese	0.56 mg	16%
Phosphorus	55.00 mg	7%
Potassium	379.75 mg	10%
Selenium	0.70 mcg	1%
Sodium	14.59 mg	1%
Zinc	0.34 mg	3%

Rice and Millet Pilaf with Almonds and Cilantro

Serving size: 190.89 g (6.73 oz-wt.)   Serves: 6

Nutrient	Value	Percent of daily nutrient allowance per serving
Basic components		0 25 50
Calories	230.56	12%
Protein	6.06 g	11%
Carbohydrates	37.76 g	13%
Dietary fiber	3.55 g	18%
Fat—Total	6.32 g	9%
Saturated fat	0.80 g	4%
Mono fat	3.51 g	16%

Rice and Millet Pilaf with Almonds and Cilantro *continued*

Nutrient	Value	Percent of daily nutrient allowance per serving
		0 25 50
Basic components *continued*		
Poly fat	1.61 g	7%
Omega-3 fatty acids	0.07 g	
Omega-6 fatty acids	1.54 g	
Vitamins		
Thiamin (B1)	0.21 mg	21%
Riboflavin (B2)	0.14 mg	12%
Niacin (B3)	2.60 mg	20%
Niacin equiv.	1.25 mg	9%
Vitamin B6	0.22 mg	14%
Biotin	4.66 mcg	7%
Vitamin C	1.27 mg	2%
Vitamin E	2.25 mg	28%
Folate	32.45 mcg	18%
Vitamin K	13.79 mcg	20%
Pantothenic acid	0.59 mg	8%
Minerals		
Calcium	35.50 mg	4%
Chromium	0.97 mcg	1%
Copper	0.33 mg	13%
Iodine	0.78 mcg	1%
Iron	1.44 mg	14%
Magnesium	88.33 mg	32%
Manganese	1.38 mg	39%
Molybdenum	1.94 mcg	1%
Phosphorus	185.67 mg	23%
Potassium	312.44 mg	8%
Selenium	5.56 mcg	10%
Sodium	316.02 mg	13%
Zinc	1.33 mg	11%

Root Stew with White Beans and Chanterelles

Serving size: 232.63 g (8.21 oz-wt.)   Serves: 8

Nutrient	Value	Percent of daily nutrient allowance per serving
		0 25 50
Basic components		
Calories	130.50	7%
Protein	4.45 g	8%
Carbohydrates	21.33 g	7%
Dietary fiber	6.65 g	33%
Fat—Total	3.77 g	6%
Saturated fat	0.54 g	2%
Mono fat	2.54 g	11%
Poly fat	0.50 g	2%
Omega-3 fatty acids	0.09 g	
Omega-6 fatty acids	0.40 g	

Root Stew with White Beans and Chanterelles *continued*

Nutrient	Value	Percent of daily nutrient allowance per serving
Vitamins		
Vitamin A	537.66 RE	67%
Thiamin (B1)	0.18 mg	18%
Riboflavin (B2)	0.09 mg	8%
Niacin (B3)	1.05 mg	8%
Niacin equiv.	0.80 mg	6%
Vitamin B6	0.23 mg	15%
Biotin	1.47 mcg	2%
Vitamin C	21.60 mg	36%
Vitamin D	0.58 mcg	12%
Vitamin E	1.16 mg	15%
Folate	81.68 mcg	45%
Vitamin K	28.53 mcg	42%
Pantothenic acid	0.64 mg	9%
Minerals		
Calcium	75.60 mg	9%
Chromium	2.29 mcg	2%
Copper	0.24 mg	10%
Iron	1.75 mg	17%
Magnesium	57.20 mg	20%
Manganese	0.39 mg	11%
Molybdenum	2.56 mcg	2%
Phosphorus	123.48 mg	15%
Potassium	665.75 mg	18%
Selenium	1.81 mcg	3%
Sodium	180.36 mg	8%
Zinc	0.94 mg	8%

Salmon Omelet with Fresh Dill

Serving size: 162.42 g (5.73 oz-wt.)   Serves: 2

Nutrient	Value	Percent of daily nutrient allowance per serving
Basic components		
Calories	238.55	12%
Protein	28.07 g	52%
Fat—Total	12.77 g	19%
Saturated fat	3.30 g	15%
Mono fat	5.29 g	24%
Poly fat	2.76 g	12%
Omega-3 fatty acids	1.37 g	
Omega-6 fatty acids	1.13 g	
Cholesterol	259.28 mg	86%
Vitamins		
Vitamin A	154.09 RE	19%
Thiamin (B1)	0.05 mg	5%
Riboflavin (B2)	0.46 mg	38%
Niacin (B3)	5.87 mg	45%
Niacin equiv.	5.33 mg	40%
Vitamin B6	0.39 mg	24%
Vitamin B12	0.82 mcg	41%
Biotin	10.02 mcg	15%

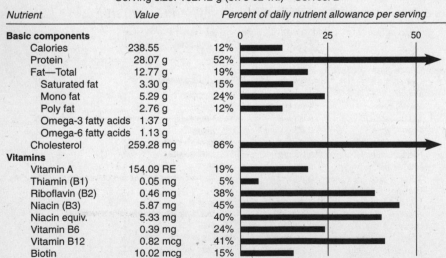

Salmon Omelet with Fresh Dill *continued*

Nutrient	Value	Percent of daily nutrient allowance per serving
Vitamins *continued*		0 25 50
Vitamin C	2.57 mg	4%
Vitamin D	6.60 mcg	132%
Vitamin E	2.24 mg	28%
Folate	34.99 mcg	19%
Vitamin K	25.00 mcg	37%
Pantothenic acid	1.22 mg	17%
Minerals		
Calcium	279.70 mg	35%
Copper	0.10 mg	4%
Iodine	26.50 mcg	18%
Iron	1.87 mg	19%
Magnesium	36.30 mg	13%
Manganese	0.05 mg	1%
Molybdenum	12.11 mcg	7%
Phosphorus	436.07 mg	55%
Potassium	469.71 mg	13%
Selenium	50.73 mcg	92%
Sodium	925.87 mg	39%
Zinc	1.64 mg	14%

Sardine Spread

Serving size: 40.85 g (1.44 oz-wt.)   Serves: 4

Nutrient	Value	Percent of daily nutrient allowance per serving
Basic components		0 25 50
Calories	91.09	5%
Protein	8.40 g	15%
Carbohydrates	1.94 g	1%
Dietary fiber	0.49 g	2%
Fat—Total	5.60 g	8%
Saturated fat	0.81 g	4%
Mono fat	1.97 g	9%
Poly fat	2.64 g	12%
Omega-3 fatty acids	0.47 g	
Omega-6 fatty acids	2.04 g	
Cholesterol	44.03 mg	15%
Vitamins		
Vitamin A	28.43 RE	4%
Thiamin (B1)	0.08 mg	8%
Riboflavin (B2)	0.09 mg	8%
Niacin (B3)	1.86 mg	14%
Niacin equiv.	1.66 mg	13%
Vitamin B6	0.07 mg	5%
Vitamin B12	2.77 mcg	139%
Biotin	0.42 mcg	1%
Vitamin C	4.28 mg	7%
Vitamin D	2.11 mcg	42%
Vitamin E	0.22 mg	3%
Folate	11.40 mcg	6%
Pantothenic acid	0.25 mg	4%

Sardine Spread *continued*

Nutrient	Value	Percent of daily nutrient allowance per serving
Minerals		0　　　　25　　　　50
Calcium	138.88 mg	17%
Copper	0.12 mg	5%
Iron	1.34 mg	13%
Magnesium	17.39 mg	6%
Manganese	0.10 mg	3%
Molybdenum	1.05 mcg	1%
Phosphorus	183.08 mg	23%
Potassium	165.34 mg	4%
Selenium	16.70 mcg	30%
Sodium	161.91 mg	7%
Zinc	0.61 mg	5%

Shrimp Potage

Serving size: 346.67 g (12.23 oz-wt.)　Serves: 2

Nutrient	Value	Percent of daily nutrient allowance per serving
Basic components		0　　　　25　　　　50
Calories	217.82	11%
Protein	9.86 g	18%
Carbohydrates	14.33 g	5%
Dietary fiber	0.99 g	5%
Fat—Total	14.05 g	21%
Saturated fat	1.94 g	9%
Mono fat	10.06 g	45%
Poly fat	1.60 g	7%
Omega-3 fatty acids	0.24 g	
Omega-6 fatty acids	1.33 g	
Cholesterol	70.19 mg	23%
Vitamins		
Vitamin A	775.81 RE	97%
Thiamin (B1)	0.07 mg	7%
Riboflavin (B2)	0.04 mg	3%
Niacin (B3)	1.33 mg	10%
Niacin equiv.	2.21 mg	17%
Vitamin B6	0.32 mg	20%
Vitamin B12	0.54 mcg	27%
Vitamin C	7.83 mg	13%
Vitamin D	1.29 mcg	26%
Vitamin E	2.13 mg	27%
Folate	24.52 mcg	14%
Pantothenic acid	0.36 mg	5%
Minerals		
Calcium	70.49 mg	9%
Copper	0.15 mg	6%
Iron	2.15 mg	21%
Magnesium	38.57 mg	14%
Manganese	0.41 mg	12%
Molybdenum	3.00 mcg	2%
Phosphorus	105.70 mg	13%
Potassium	420.43 mg	11%

Shrimp Potage *continued*

Nutrient	Value	Percent of daily nutrient allowance per serving
Minerals *continued*		
Selenium	18.10 mcg	33%
Sodium	722.21 mg	30%
Zinc	1.42 mg	12%

Simple Roast Chicken

Serving size: 240.00 g (8.47 oz-wt.)   Serves: 4

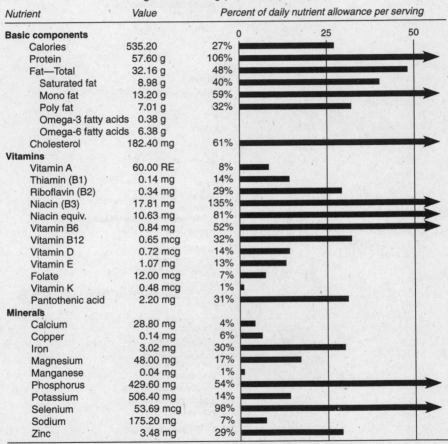

Nutrient	Value	Percent of daily nutrient allowance per serving
Basic components		
Calories	535.20	27%
Protein	57.60 g	106%
Fat—Total	32.16 g	48%
Saturated fat	8.98 g	40%
Mono fat	13.20 g	59%
Poly fat	7.01 g	32%
Omega-3 fatty acids	0.38 g	
Omega-6 fatty acids	6.38 g	
Cholesterol	182.40 mg	61%
Vitamins		
Vitamin A	60.00 RE	8%
Thiamin (B1)	0.14 mg	14%
Riboflavin (B2)	0.34 mg	29%
Niacin (B3)	17.81 mg	135%
Niacin equiv.	10.63 mg	81%
Vitamin B6	0.84 mg	52%
Vitamin B12	0.65 mcg	32%
Vitamin D	0.72 mcg	14%
Vitamin E	1.07 mg	13%
Folate	12.00 mcg	7%
Vitamin K	0.48 mcg	1%
Pantothenic acid	2.20 mg	31%
Minerals		
Calcium	28.80 mg	4%
Copper	0.14 mg	6%
Iron	3.02 mg	30%
Magnesium	48.00 mg	17%
Manganese	0.04 mg	1%
Phosphorus	429.60 mg	54%
Potassium	506.40 mg	14%
Selenium	53.69 mcg	98%
Sodium	175.20 mg	7%
Zinc	3.48 mg	29%

Sesame Seaweed Sprinkle (Wakame Gomashio)
Serving size: 10.00 g (0.35 oz-wt.)   Serves: 1

Nutrient	Value	Percent of daily nutrient allowance per serving
Minerals		
Calcium	110.40 mg	14%
Magnesium	37.30 mg	13%
Potassium	119.60 mg	3%
Sodium	91.90 mg	4%
Zinc	0.46 mg	4%

Spanish Fish Soup
Serving size: 237.76 g (8.39 oz-wt.)   Serves: 8

Nutrient	Value	Percent of daily nutrient allowance per serving
Basic components		
Calories	149.17	7%
Protein	22.08 g	41%
Carbohydrates	3.64 g	1%
Dietary fiber	0.28 g	1%
Fat—Total	4.59 g	7%
Saturated fat	0.80 g	4%
Mono fat	2.67 g	12%
Poly fat	0.90 g	4%
Omega-3 fatty acids	0.44 g	
Omega-6 fatty acids	0.36 g	
Cholesterol	106.59 mg	36%
Vitamins		
Vitamin A	33.52 RE	4%
Thiamin (B1)	0.08 mg	8%
Riboflavin (B2)	0.22 mg	18%
Niacin (B3)	2.50 mg	19%
Niacin equiv.	4.12 mg	31%
Vitamin B6	0.24 mg	15%
Vitamin B12	11.20 mcg	560%
Biotin	0.48 mcg	1%
Vitamin C	7.00 mg	12%
Vitamin D	0.67 mcg	13%
Vitamin E	1.46 mg	18%
Folate	16.22 mcg	9%
Vitamin K	0.40 mcg	1%
Pantothenic acid	0.36 mg	5%
Minerals		
Calcium	46.42 mg	6%
Chromium	2.13 mcg	2%
Copper	0.65 mg	26%
Iron	3.37 mg	34%
Magnesium	50.79 mg	18%
Manganese	0.18 mg	5%
Phosphorus	280.12 mg	35%
Potassium	556.14 mg	15%
Selenium	54.04 mcg	98%
Sodium	415.30 mg	17%
Zinc	1.45 mg	12%

Stir-fried Bok Choy with Shrimp

Serving size: 119.78 g (4.23 oz-wt.)   Serves: 4

Nutrient	Value	Percent of daily nutrient allowance per serving
Basic components		
Calories	71.69	4%
Protein	6.51 g	12%
Carbohydrates	3.36 g	1%
Dietary fiber	1.48 g	7%
Fat—Total	3.92 g	6%
Saturated fat	0.56 g	3%
Mono fat	2.58 g	12%
Poly fat	0.63 g	3%
Omega-3 fatty acids	0.21 g	
Omega-6 fatty acids	0.38 g	
Cholesterol	31.92 mg	11%
Vitamins		
Vitamin A	223.78 RE	28%
Thiamin (B1)	0.05 mg	5%
Riboflavin (B2)	0.08 mg	6%
Niacin (B3)	1.29 mg	10%
Niacin equiv.	1.48 mg	11%
Vitamin B6	0.20 mg	13%
Vitamin B12	0.24 mcg	12%
Biotin	1.62 mcg	2%
Vitamin C	33.63 mg	56%
Vitamin D	0.80 mcg	16%
Vitamin E	0.71 mg	9%
Folate	52.44 mcg	29%
Vitamin K	12.94 mcg	19%
Pantothenic acid	0.17 mg	2%
Calcium	93.81 mg	12%
Chromium	0.97 mcg	1%
Copper	0.10 mg	4%
Iron	1.42 mg	14%
Magnesium	26.91 mg	10%
Manganese	0.21 mg	6%
Phosphorus	85.64 mg	11%
Potassium	262.78 mg	7%
Selenium	8.39 mcg	15%
Sodium	580.96 mg	24%
Zinc	0.46 mg	4%

Sunflower Seed Soup

Serving size: 278.93 g (9.84 oz-wt.)   Serves: 6

Nutrient	Value	Percent of daily nutrient allowance per serving
Basic components		
Calories	104.61	5%
Protein	3.04 g	6%
Carbohydrates	10.59 g	4%
Dietary fiber	3.27 g	16%
Fat—Total	6.54 g	10%

Sunflower Seed Soup *continued*

Nutrient	Value	Percent of daily nutrient allowance per serving

Basic components *continued*

Nutrient	Value	Percent
Saturated fat	0.71 g	3%
Mono fat	1.24 g	6%
Poly fat	4.28 g	19%
Omega-3 fatty acids	0.02 g	
Omega-6 fatty acids	4.25 g	

Vitamins

Nutrient	Value	Percent
Vitamin A	675.14 RE	84%
Thiamin (B1)	0.09 mg	9%
Riboflavin (B2)	0.07 mg	6%
Niacin (B3)	1.01 mg	8%
Niacin equiv.	0.63 mg	5%
Vitamin B6	0.22 mg	13%
Vitamin B12	0 mcg	0%
Biotin	1.86 mcg	3%
Vitamin C	9.27 mg	15%
Vitamin E	6.09 mg	76%
Folate	37.75 mcg	21%
Vitamin K	35.18 mcg	52%
Pantothenic acid	1.00 mg	14%

Minerals

Nutrient	Value	Percent
Calcium	40.92 mg	5%
Chromium	2.84 mcg	2%
Copper	0.27 mg	11%
Iron	1.21 mg	12%
Magnesium	33.02 mg	12%
Manganese	0.37 mg	11%
Molybdenum	2.93 mcg	2%
Phosphorus	184.73 mg	23%
Potassium	371.51 mg	10%
Selenium	13.39 mcg	24%
Sodium	478.25 mg	20%
Zinc	0.98 mg	8%

Winter Lunch

Serving size: 558.50 g (19.70 oz-wt.)   Serves: 1

Amount per serving	Food item
12 oz-wt	Chicken Soup
4.7 oz-wt	Tart with Greens and Leeks
3 oz-wt	Cucumber-Radish Salad with Wakame and Walnut-Lime Dressing

Nutrients per serving

Calories	392.46
Protein	17.07 g
Carbohydrates	26.31 g
Dietary fiber	5.21 g
Percent calories from fat	57%
Fat—Total	25.38 g
Saturated fat	5.69 g

Winter Lunch *continued*

Nutrients per serving

Vitamin A	1008.96 RE
Vitamin C	39.13 mg
Percent calories from carbohydrates	26%

Nutrient	Value	Percent of daily nutrient allowance per serving
Basic components		
Calories	392.46	20%
Protein	17.07 g	31%
Carbohydrates	26.31 g	9%
Dietary fiber	5.21 g	26%
Fat—Total	25.38 g	38%
Saturated fat	5.69 g	26%
Mono fat	11.76 g	53%
Poly fat	6.33 g	28%
Omega-3 fatty acids	1.70 g	
Omega-6 fatty acids	4.63 g	
Cholesterol	154.71 mg	52%
Vitamins		
Vitamin A	1008.96 RE	126%
Thiamin (B1)	0.24 mg	24%
Riboflavin (B2)	0.42 mg	35%
Niacin (B3)	3.97 mg	30%
Niacin equiv.	4.26 mg	32%
Vitamin B6	0.40 mg	25%
Vitamin B12	0.50 mcg	25%
Biotin	8.20 mcg	13%
Vitamin C	39.13 mg	65%
Vitamin D	0.52 mcg	10%
Vitamin E	4.44 mg	55%
Folate	75.90 mcg	42%
Vitamin K	118.33 mcg	174%
Pantothenic acid	1.49 mg	21%
Minerals		
Calcium	243.83 mg	30%
Copper	0.24 mg	10%
Iodine	15.92 mcg	11%
Iron	3.49 mg	35%
Magnesium	102.97 mg	37%
Manganese	1.36 mg	39%
Molybdenum	12.11 mcg	7%
Phosphorus	303.42 mg	38%
Potassium	781.28 mg	21%
Selenium	31.64 mcg	58%
Sodium	673.91 mg	28%
Zinc	2.70 mg	22%

Winter Dinner

Serving size: 731.20 g (25.79 oz-wt.)   Serves: 1

Amount per serving	Food item
8 oz-wt	Miso Soup with Wild Mushrooms and Garlic
4 oz-wt	Poached Red Snapper
2 oz-wt	Parsley Sauce
3 oz-wt	Puree of Yams
1/2 cup	Medium Grain Brown Rice-Cooked
10 g	Sesame Seaweed Sprinkle (Wakame Gomashio)
5 oz-wt	Broiled Bananas

Nutrients per serving

Calories	750.58
Protein	46.70 g
Carbohydrates	104.56 g
Dietary fiber	13.72 g
Percent calories from fat	20%
Fat—Total	17.33 g
Saturated fat	7.16 g
Vitamin A	1591.77 RE
Vitamin C	30.19 mg
Percent calories from carbohydrates	55%

Nutrient	Value	Percent of daily nutrient allowance per serving
Basic components		
Calories	750.58	38%
Protein	46.70 g	86%
Carbohydrates	104.56 g	36%
Dietary fiber	13.72 g	69%
Fat—Total	17.33 g	26%
Saturated fat	7.16 g	32%
Mono fat	4.26 g	19%
Poly fat	4.71 g	21%
Cholesterol	83.36 mg	28%
Vitamins		
Vitamin A	1591.77 RE	199%
Thiamin (B1)	0.39 mg	39%
Riboflavin (B2)	0.45 mg	37%
Niacin (B3)	4.86 mg	37%
Niacin equiv.	6.36 mg	48%
Vitamin B6	1.58 mg	99%
Vitamin B12	0.34 mcg	17%
Biotin	6.80 mcg	10%
Vitamin C	30.19 mg	50%
Vitamin D	0.17 mcg	3%
Vitamin E	2.00 mg	25%
Folate	58.93 mcg	33%
Vitamin K	10.07 mcg	15%
Pantothenic acid	2.20 mg	31%
Minerals		
Calcium	219.14 mg	27%
Chromium	0.62 mcg	0%

Winter Dinner *continued*

Nutrient	Value	Percent of daily nutrient allowance per serving
Minerals *continued*		
Copper	0.50 mg	20%
Iodine	11.00 mcg	7%
Iron	9.87 mg	99%
Magnesium	206.88 mg	74%
Manganese	2.30 mg	66%
Phosphorus	464.95 mg	58%
Potassium	1398.18 mg	37%
Selenium	11.62 mcg	21%
Sodium	1121.95 mg	47%
Zinc	3.48 mg	29%

Winter—Whole Day

Serving size: 1522.40 g (53.70 oz-wt.)   Serves: 1

Amount per serving	Food item
8 oz-wt	Creamy Millet Breakfast Porridge
19.7 oz-wt	Winter Lunch
26 oz-wt	Winter Dinner

Nutrients per serving

Calories	1369.93
Protein	70.58 g
Carbohydrates	158.80 g
Dietary fiber	22.85 g
Percent calories from fat	34%
Fat—Total	53.23 g
Saturated fat	13.99 g
Vitamin A	2613.63 RE
Vitamin C	70.98 mg
Percent calories from carbohydrates	45%

Nutrient	Value	Percent of daily nutrient allowance per serving
Basic components		
Calories	1369.93	69%
Protein	70.58 g	130%
Carbohydrates	158.80 g	55%
Dietary fiber	22.85 g	114%
Fat—Total	53.23 g	80%
Saturated fat	13.99 g	63%
Mono fat	19.59 g	88%
Poly fat	16.47 g	74%
Omega-3 fatty acids	5.38 g	
Omega-6 fatty acids	10.01 g	
Cholesterol	238.74 mg	80%
Vitamins		
Vitamin A	2613.63 RE	327%
Thiamin (B1)	0.76 mg	76%
Riboflavin (B2)	1.05 mg	88%
Niacin (B3)	10.82 mg	82%

Winter—Whole Day *continued*

Nutrient	Value		Percent of daily nutrient allowance per serving
Vitamins *continued*			0 25 50
Niacin equiv.	11.99 mg	91%	
Vitamin B6	2.15 mg	134%	
Vitamin B12	0.84 mcg	42%	
Biotin	18.90 mcg	29%	
Vitamin C	70.98 mg	118%	
Vitamin D	0.69 mcg	14%	
Vitamin E	11.86 mg	148%	
Folate	176.54 mcg	98%	
Vitamin K	128.65 mcg	189%	
Pantothenic acid	4.47 mg	64%	
Minerals			
Calcium	499.51 mg	62%	
Copper	1.19 mg	47%	
Iodine	27.61 mcg	18%	
Iron	15.91 mg	159%	
Magnesium	392.74 mg	140%	
Manganese	4.60 mg	131%	
Molybdenum	13.88 mcg	9%	
Phosphorus	988.46 mg	124%	
Potassium	2440.27 mg	65%	
Selenium	48.09 mcg	87%	
Sodium	2029.67 mg	85%	
Zinc	7.58 mg	63%	

Winter—Meatless Lunch

Serving size: 538.65 g (19.00 oz-wt.)   Serves: 1

Amount per serving	Food item
12 oz-wt	Root Stew with White Beans and Chanterelles
3 oz-wt	Curried Mustard Greens with Parmesan
4 oz-wt	Plain Kasha

Nutrients per serving

Calories	350.12
Protein	13.43 g
Carbohydrates	53.74 g
Dietary fiber	14.59 g
Percent calories from fat	28%
Fat—Total	11.44 g
Saturated fat	4.09 g
Vitamin A	1184.77 RE
Vitamin C	79.14 mg
Percent calories from carbohydrates	58%

Nutrient	Value		Percent of daily nutrient allowance per serving
Basic components			0 25 50
Calories	350.12	18%	
Protein	13.43 g	25%	

Winter—Meatless Lunch *continued*

Nutrient	Value	Percent of daily nutrient allowance per serving
Basic components *continued*		0 25 50
Carbohydrates	53.74 g	19%
Dietary fiber	14.59 g	73%
Fat—Total	11.44 g	17%
Saturated fat	4.09 g	18%
Mono fat	5.46 g	25%
Poly fat	1.19 g	5%
Omega-3 fatty acids	0.23 g	
Omega-6 fatty acids	0.96 g	
Cholesterol	12.66 mg	4%
Vitamins		
Vitamin A	1184.77 RE	148%
Thiamin (B1)	0.35 mg	35%
Riboflavin (B2)	0.34 mg	28%
Niacin (B3)	3.92 mg	30%
Niacin equiv.	2.67 mg	20%
Vitamin B6	0.54 mg	34%
Vitamin B12	0.05 mcg	3%
Biotin	2.27 mcg	3%
Vitamin C	79.14 mg	132%
Vitamin D	0.95 mcg	19%
Vitamin E	3.47 mg	43%
Folate	253.54 mcg	141%
Vitamin K	152.20 mcg	230%
Pantothenic acid	1.42 mg	20%
Minerals		
Calcium	243.47 mg	30%
Chromium	3.35 mcg	3%
Copper	0.74 mg	30%
Iron	4.17 mg	42%
Magnesium	172.69 mg	62%
Manganese	1.26 mg	36%
Molybdenum	7.29 mcg	4%
Phosphorus	332.22 mg	42%
Potassium	1448.57 mg	39%
Selenium	3.82 mcg	7%
Sodium	627.56 mg	26%
Zinc	2.43 mg	20%

Winter—Meatless Dinner

Serving size: 871.80 g (30.75 oz-wt.)   Serves: 1

Amount per serving	Food item
1½ cup	Vegetarian Vegetable Soup with Water
5 oz-wt	Anasazi Beans with Collards and Shiitake
6 oz-wt	Flavorful Rice and Barley
3 oz-wt	Carrots-Fresh Slices-Boiled-Cup
4 oz-wt	Almond Milk Pudding

Winter—Meatless Dinner *continued*

Nutrients per serving

Calories	684.65
Protein	20.33 g
Carbohydrates	117.92 g
Dietary fiber	20.06 g
Percent calories from fat	22%
Fat—Total	16.94 g
Saturated fat	2.08 g
Vitamin A	2582.82 RE
Vitamin C	26.07 mg
Percent calories from carbohydrates	67%

Nutrient	Value		Percent of daily nutrient allowance per serving
Basic components			
Calories	684.65	34%	
Protein	20.33 g	37%	
Carbohydrates	117.92 g	41%	
Dietary fiber	20.06 g	100%	
Fat—Total	16.94 g	25%	
Saturated fat	2.08 g	9%	
Mono fat	9.65 g	43%	
Poly fat	4.19 g	19%	
Omega-3 fatty acids	0.30 g		
Omega-6 fatty acids	3.81 g		
Vitamins			
Vitamin A	2582.82 RE	323%	
Thiamin (B1)	0.58 mg	58%	
Riboflavin (B2)	0.50 mg	41%	
Niacin (B3)	5.64 mg	43%	
Niacin equiv.	4.15 mg	31%	
Vitamin B6	0.74 mg	46%	
Vitamin B12	0 mcg	0%	
Biotin	16.32 mcg	25%	
Vitamin C	26.07 mg	43%	
Vitamin D	1.08 mcg	22%	
Vitamin E	8.17 mg	102%	
Folate	197.32 mcg	110%	
Vitamin K	16.22 mcg	24%	
Pantothenic acid	2.14 mg	31%	
Minerals			
Calcium	197.40 mg	25%	
Chromium	3.25 mcg	3%	
Copper	1.06 mg	42%	
Iodine	2.12 mcg	1%	
Iron	6.76 mg	68%	
Magnesium	204.46 mg	73%	
Manganese	4.06 mg	116%	
Molybdenum	77.88 mcg	48%	
Phosphorus	462.61 mg	58%	
Potassium	1436.52 mg	38%	
Selenium	26.21 mcg	48%	
Sodium	1738.02 mg	72%	
Zinc	4.48 mg	37%	

Winter—Whole Day Meatless

Serving size: 1615.95 g (57.00 oz-wt.)   Serves: 1

Amount per serving	Food item
8 oz-wt	Creamy Whole-Grain Breakfast Porridge
19 oz-wt	Winter—Meatless Lunch
30 oz-wt	Winter—Meatless Dinner

Nutrients per serving

Calories	1238.88
Protein	39.70 g
Carbohydrates	195.87 g
Dietary fiber	37.97 g
Percent calories from fat	27%
Fat—Total	38.34 g
Saturated fat	7.19 g
Vitamin A	3704.53 RE
Vitamin C	105.98 mg
Percent calories from carbohydrates	61%

Nutrient	Value	Percent of daily nutrient allowance per serving
Basic components		
Calories	1238.88	62%
Protein	39.70 g	73%
Carbohydrates	195.87 g	68%
Dietary fiber	37.97 g	190%
Fat—Total	38.34 g	58%
Saturated fat	7.19 g	32%
Mono fat	18.41 g	83%
Poly fat	10.67 g	48%
Omega-3 fatty acids	2.12 g	
Omega-6 fatty acids	8.50 g	
Cholesterol	12.66 mg	4%
Vitamins		
Vitamin A	3704.53 RE	463%
Thiamin (B1)	1.05 mg	105%
Riboflavin (B2)	1.00 mg	83%
Niacin (B3)	11.38 mg	86%
Niacin equiv.	8.03 mg	61%
Vitamin B6	1.42 mg	89%
Vitamin B12	0.05 mcg	3%
Biotin	22.04 mcg	34%
Vitamin C	105.98 mg	177%
Vitamin D	2.00 mcg	40%
Vitamin E	16.85 mg	211%
Folate	487.26 mcg	271%
Vitamin K	172.18 mcg	253%
Pantothenic acid	4.28 mg	61%
Minerals		
Calcium	470.82 mg	59%
Chromium	6.52 mcg	5%
Copper	2.22 mg	89%
Iodine	3.10 mcg	2%
Iron	13.24 mg	132%
Magnesium	453.38 mg	162%

Winter—Whole Day Meatless *continued*

Nutrient	Value	Percent of daily nutrient allowance per serving

Minerals *continued*

			0	25	50
Manganese	6.14 mg	175%			
Molybdenum	85.03 mcg	52%			
Phosphorus	999.86 mg	125%			
Potassium	3099.52 mg	83%			
Selenium	34.12 mcg	62%			
Sodium	2547.88 mg	106%			
Zinc	8.17 mg	68%			

Summer Breakfast

Serving size: 340.20 g (12.00 oz-wt.)   Serves: 1

Amount per serving	Food item
8 oz-wt	Fresh Fruit Salad with Toasted Sunflower Seeds
4 oz-wt	Oat-Dulse Crackers

Nutrients per serving

Calories	600.96
Protein	16.70 g
Carbohydrates	64.88 g
Dietary fiber	12.39 g
Percent calories from fat	49%
Fat—Total	34.55 g
Saturated fat	8.58 g
Vitamin A	115.85 RE
Vitamin C	38.57 mg
Percent Calories from carbohydrates	41%

Nutrient	Value	Percent of daily nutrient allowance per serving

Basic components

			0	25	50
Calories	600.96	30%			
Protein	16.70 g	31%			
Carbohydrates	64.88 g	22%			
Dietary fiber	12.39 g	62%			
Fat—Total	34.55 g	52%			
Saturated fat	8.58 g	39%			
Mono fat	7.72 g	35%			
Poly fat	16.34 g	74%			
Cholesterol	24.73 mg	8%			

Vitamins

			0	25	50
Vitamin A	115.85 RE	14%			
Thiamin (B1)	0.91 mg	91%			
Riboflavin (B2)	0.27 mg	23%			
Niacin (B3)	4.09 mg	31%			
Niacin equiv.	3.08 mg	23%			
Vitamin B6	0.65 mg	41%			
Vitamin B12	0.01 mcg	1%			
Biotin	8.48 mcg	13%			
Vitamin C	38.57 mg	64%			

Summer Breakfast *continued*

Nutrient	Value	Percent of daily nutrient allowance per serving
Vitamins *continued*		
Vitamin D	0.16 mcg	3%
Vitamin E	11.88 mg	149%
Folate	147.77 mcg	82%
Vitamin K	139.02 mcg	204%
Pantothenic acid	3.90 mg	56%
Minerals		
Calcium	98.55 mg	12%
Copper	1.07 mg	43%
Iodine	2.95 mcg	2%
Iron	4.57 mg	46%
Magnesium	186.53 mg	67%
Manganese	2.66 mg	76%
Phosphorus	611.61 mg	76%
Potassium	846.87 mg	23%
Selenium	51.29 mcg	93%
Sodium	184.98 mg	8%
Zinc	3.74 mg	31%

Summer Lunch

Serving size: 367.50 g (12.96 oz-wt.)   Serves: 1

Amount per serving	Food item
6 oz-wt	Salmon Omelet with Fresh Dill
4 oz-wt	Broccoli with Mushrooms
2 pieces	Whole Wheat Bread-Toasted

Nutrients per serving

Calories	565.52
Protein	40.24 g
Carbohydrates	54.49 g
Dietary fiber	8.46 g
Percent calories from fat	34%
Fat—Total	21.89 g
Saturated fat	4.69 g
Vitamin A	287.76 RE
Vitamin C	80.54 mg
Percent calories from carbohydrates	38%

Nutrient	Value	Percent of daily nutrient allowance per serving
Basic components		
Calories	565.52	28%
Protein	40.24 g	74%
Carbohydrates	54.49 g	19%
Dietary fiber	8.46 g	42%
Fat—Total	21.89 g	33%
Saturated fat	4.69 g	21%
Mono fat	8.95 g	40%

Summer Lunch *continued*

Nutrient	Value	Percent of daily nutrient allowance per serving
Basic components *continued*		
Poly fat	6.10 g	27%
Cholesterol	271.53 mg	91%
Vitamins		
Vitamin A	287.76 RE	36%
Thiamin (B1)	0.36 mg	36%
Riboflavin (B2)	0.89 mg	74%
Niacin (B3)	11.08 mg	84%
Niacin equiv.	8.07 mg	61%
Vitamin B6	0.75 mg	47%
Vitamin B12	0.86 mcg	43%
Biotin	21.18 mcg	33%
Vitamin C	80.54 mg	134%
Vitamin D	7.53 mcg	151%
Vitamin E	5.52 mg	69%
Folate	130.77 mcg	73%
Vitamin K	194.42 mcg	286%
Pantothenic acid	2.59 mg	37%
Minerals		
Calcium	366.49 mg	46%
Chromium	1.85 mcg	1%
Copper	0.51 mg	20%
Iodine	30.19 mcg	20%
Iron	5.90 mg	59%
Magnesium	136.29 mg	49%
Manganese	2.03 mg	58%
Molybdenum	18.11 mcg	11%
Phosphorus	712.71 mg	89%
Potassium	1151.88 mg	31%
Selenium	95.75 mcg	174%
Sodium	1448.66 mg	60%
Zinc	3.64 mg	30%

Summer Dinner

Serving size: 662.23 g (23.36 oz-wt.)   Serves: 1

Amount per serving	Food item
8 oz-wt	Cucumber-Avocado Soup
6 oz-wt	Stir-fried Bok Choy with Shrimp
5	Baby Carrots
4 oz-wt	Polenta
2 Tbs	Blanched Slivered Almonds
3 oz-wt	Apple-Strawberry Mold

Nutrients per serving

Calories	378.20
Protein	16.75 g
Carbohydrates	34.23 g
Dietary fiber	8.16 g
Percent calories from fat	50%

Summer Dinner *continued*

Nutrients per serving continued

Fat—Total	22.63 g
Saturated fat	2.89 g
Vitamin A	472.43 RE
Vitamin C	68.26 mg
Percent calories from carbohydrates	34%

Nutrient	Value	Percent of daily nutrient allowance per serving
Basic components		
Calories	378.20	19%
Protein	16.75 g	31%
Carbohydrates	34.23 g	12%
Dietary fiber	8.16 g	41%
Fat—Total	22.63 g	34%
Saturated fat	2.89 g	13%
Mono fat	13.47 g	61%
Poly fat	3.78 g	17%
Cholesterol	46.95 mg	16%
Vitamins		
Vitamin A	472.43 RE	59%
Thiamin (B1)	0.20 mg	20%
Riboflavin (B2)	0.34 mg	29%
Niacin (B3)	3.95 mg	30%
Niacin equiv.	2.51 mg	19%
Vitamin B6	0.54 mg	34%
Vitamin B12	0.35 mcg	17%
Biotin	4.65 mcg	7%
Vitamin C	68.26 mg	114%
Vitamin D	1.14 mcg	23%
Vitamin E	2.09 mg	26%
Folate	143.76 mcg	80%
Vitamin K	31.04 mcg	46%
Pantothenic acid	0.99 mg	14%
Minerals		
Calcium	234.74 mg	29%
Chromium	1.38 mcg	1%
Copper	0.53 mg	21%
Iodine	1.54 mcg	1%
Iron	4.71 mg	47%
Magnesium	155.48 mg	56%
Manganese	0.73 mg	21%
Molybdenum	8.35 mcg	5%
Phosphorus	311.07 mg	39%
Potassium	1224.19 mg	33%
Selenium	30.15 mcg	55%
Sodium	926.31 mg	39%
Zinc	2.17 mg	18%

Summer—Whole Day

Serving size: 1360.80 g (48.00 oz-wt.)   Serves: 1

Amount per serving	Food item
12 oz-wt	Summer Breakfast
13 oz-wt	Summer Lunch
23 oz-wt	Summer Dinner

Nutrients per serving

Calories	1460.34
Protein	72.31 g
Carbohydrates	148.95 g
Dietary fiber	28.81 g
Percent calories from fat	43%
Fat—Total	72.84 g
Saturated fat	15.60 g
Vitamin A	972.77 RE
Vitamin C	203.02 mg
Percent Calories from carbohydrates	39%

Nutrient	Value	Percent of daily nutrient allowance per serving
Basic components		
Calories	1460.34	73%
Protein	72.31 g	133%
Carbohydrates	148.95 g	51%
Dietary fiber	28.81 g	144%
Fat—Total	72.84 g	109%
Saturated fat	15.60 g	70%
Mono fat	26.20 g	118%
Poly fat	24.73 g	111%
Omega-3 fatty acids	2.92 g	
Omega-6 fatty acids	22.57 g	
Cholesterol	352.60 mg	118%
Vitamins		
Vitamin A	972.77 RE	122%
Thiamin (B1)	1.47 mg	147%
Riboflavin (B2)	1.44 mg	120%
Niacin (B3)	19.27 mg	146%
Niacin equiv.	14.14 mg	107%
Vitamin B6	2.03 mg	127%
Vitamin B12	1.30 mcg	65%
Biotin	35.42 mcg	54%
Vitamin C	203.02 mg	338%
Vitamin D	9.10 mcg	182%
Vitamin E	19.93 mg	249%
Folate	446.38 mcg	248%
Vitamin K	372.05 mcg	547%
Pantothenic acid	7.67 mg	110%
Minerals		
Calcium	697.59 mg	87%
Chromium	3.54 mcg	3%
Copper	1.98 mg	79%
Iodine	35.12 mcg	23%
Iron	15.36 mg	154%
Magnesium	444.52 mg	159%

Summer—Whole Day *continued*

Nutrient	Value	Percent of daily nutrient allowance per serving
Minerals *continued*		0 25 50
Manganese	5.58 mg	159%
Molybdenum	28.48 mcg	17%
Phosphorus	1589.34 mg	199%
Potassium	3276.53 mg	87%
Selenium	182.23 mcg	331%
Sodium	2684.83 mg	112%
Zinc	9.18 mg	77%

Summer—Meatless Lunch

Serving size: 385.53 g (13.60 oz-wt.)   Serves 1

Amount per serving	Food item
2	Yellow Corn-on-the-Cob-Boiled
8 oz-wt	Chickpea Taboulleh
1 tsp	Unsalted Butter

Nutrients per serving

Calories	570.83
Protein	18.61 g
Carbohydrates	83.22 g
Dietary fiber	17.46 g
Percent calories from fat	34%
Fat—Total	22.82 g
Saturated fat	4.47 g
Vitamin A	172.50 RE
Vitamin C	43.76 mg
Percent calories from carbohydrates	54%

Nutrient	Value	Percent of daily nutrient allowance per serving
Basic components		0 25 50
Calories	570.83	29%
Protein	18.61 g	34%
Carbohydrates	83.22 g	29%
Dietary fiber	17.46 g	87%
Fat—Total	22.82 g	34%
Saturated fat	4.47g	20%
Mono fat	8.75 g	39%
Poly fat	8.17 g	37%
Cholesterol	10.36 mg	3%
Vitamins		
Vitamin A	172.50 RE	22%
Thiamin (B1)	0.67 mg	67%
Riboflavin (B2)	0.28 mg	23%
Niacin (B3)	3.79 mg	29%
Niacin equiv.	2.84 mg	22%
Vitamin B6	0.51 mg	32%
Vitamin B12	0.01 mcg	0%
Biotin	1.78 mcg	3%

Summer—Meatless Lunch *continued*

Nutrient	Value	Percent of daily nutrient allowance per serving
Vitamins *continued*		
Vitamin C	43.76 mg	73%
Vitamin D	0.07 mcg	1%
Vitamin E	4.12 mg	51%
Folate	465.20 mcg	258%
Vitamin K	1.01 mcg	1%
Pantothenic acid	2.51 mg	36%
Minerals		
Calcium	114.65 mg	14%
Chromium	7.80 mcg	6%
Copper	0.68 mg	27%
Iodine	1.01 mcg	1%
Iron	6.25 mg	62%
Magnesium	143.03 mg	51%
Manganese	1.79 mg	51%
Molybdenum	2.63 mcg	2%
Phosphorus	418.96 mg	52%
Potassium	1209.63 mg	32%
Selenium	6.76 mcg	12%
Sodium	436.45 mg	18%
Zinc	3.35 mg	28%

Summer—Meatless Dinner

Serving size: 539.42 g (19.03 oz-wt.)   Serves: 1

Amount per serving	Food item
4 oz-wt	Composed Salad with Beets and Avocado
6 oz-wt	Flavorful Rice and Barley
3 oz-wt	Miso-broiled Tofu
2½ oz-wt	Asparagus with Slivered Almonds
2	Fresh Figs

Nutrients per serving

Calories	551.97
Protein	23.59 g
Carbohydrates	72.59 g
Dietary fiber	15.81 g
Percent calories from fat	34%
Fat—Total	22.44 g
Saturated fat	3.03 g
Vitamin A	166.47 RE
Vitamin C	19.39 mg
Percent calories from carbohydrates	49%

Nutrient	Value	Percent of daily nutrient allowance per serving
Basic components		
Calories	551.97	28%
Protein	23.59 g	43%
Carbohydrates	72.59 g	25%

Summer—Meatless Dinner *continued*

Nutrient	Value	Percent of daily nutrient allowance per serving

Basic components *continued*

Nutrient	Value	Percent
Dietary fiber	15.81 g	79%
Fat—Total	22.44 g	34%
Saturated fat	3.03 g	14%
Mono fat	10.98 g	49%
Poly fat	6.61 g	30%

Vitamins

Nutrient	Value	Percent
Vitamin A	166.47 RE	21%
Thiamin (B1)	0.61 mg	61%
Riboflavin (B2)	0.46 mg	38%
Niacin (B3)	5.18 mg	39%
Niacin equiv.	5.06 mg	38%
Vitamin (B6)	0.64 mg	40%
Biotin	2.07 mcg	3%
Vitamin C	19.39 mg	32%
Vitamin E	3.26 mg	41%
Folate	237.86 mcg	132%
Vitamin K	45.31 mcg	67%
Pantothenic acid	1.50 mg	21%

Minerals

Nutrient	Value	Percent
Calcium	276.15 mg	35%
Chromium	3.25 mcg	3%
Copper	0.89 mg	36%
Iodine	2.62 mcg	2%
Iron	11.66 mg	117%
Magnesium	230.43 mg	82%
Manganese	2.91 mg	83%
Molybdenum	10.74 mcg	7%
Phosphorus	435.73 mg	54%
Potassium	1381.67 mg	37%
Selenium	19.81 mcg	36%
Sodium	542.78 mg	23%
Zinc	3.74 mg	31%

Summer—Whole Day Meatless

Serving size: 1275.75 g (45.00 oz-wt.)   Serves: 1

Amount per serving	Food item
12 oz-wt	Summer Breakfast
14 oz-wt	Summer—Meatless Lunch
19 oz-wt	Summer—Meatless Dinner

Nutrients per serving

Calories	1729.31
Protein	58.69 g
Carbohydrates	224.36 g
Dietary fiber	45.47 g
Percent calories from fat	39%
Fat—Total	79.37 g
Saturated fat	16.48 g
Vitamin A	459.22 RE
Vitamin C	100.42 mg

Summer—Whole Day Meatless *continued*

Nutrients per serving continued

Percent calories from
carbohydrates   49%

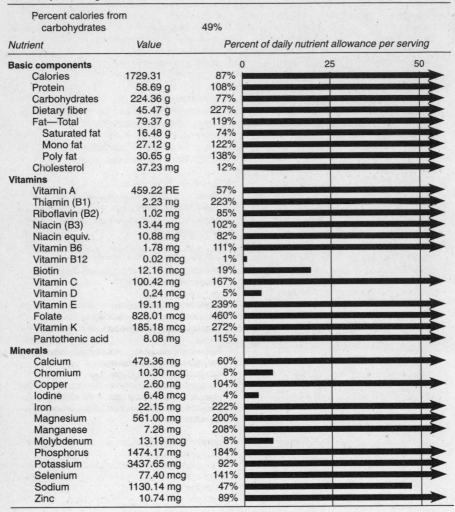

Nutrient	Value	Percent of daily nutrient allowance per serving
Basic components		
Calories	1729.31	87%
Protein	58.69 g	108%
Carbohydrates	224.36 g	77%
Dietary fiber	45.47 g	227%
Fat—Total	79.37 g	119%
Saturated fat	16.48 g	74%
Mono fat	27.12 g	122%
Poly fat	30.65 g	138%
Cholesterol	37.23 mg	12%
Vitamins		
Vitamin A	459.22 RE	57%
Thiamin (B1)	2.23 mg	223%
Riboflavin (B2)	1.02 mg	85%
Niacin (B3)	13.44 mg	102%
Niacin equiv.	10.88 mg	82%
Vitamin B6	1.78 mg	111%
Vitamin B12	0.02 mcg	1%
Biotin	12.16 mcg	19%
Vitamin C	100.42 mg	167%
Vitamin D	0.24 mcg	5%
Vitamin E	19.11 mg	239%
Folate	828.01 mcg	460%
Vitamin K	185.18 mcg	272%
Pantothenic acid	8.08 mg	115%
Minerals		
Calcium	479.36 mg	60%
Chromium	10.30 mcg	8%
Copper	2.60 mg	104%
Iodine	6.48 mcg	4%
Iron	22.15 mg	222%
Magnesium	561.00 mg	200%
Manganese	7.28 mg	208%
Molybdenum	13.19 mcg	8%
Phosphorus	1474.17 mg	184%
Potassium	3437.65 mg	92%
Selenium	77.40 mcg	141%
Sodium	1130.14 mg	47%
Zinc	10.74 mg	89%

Chicken Dinner

Serving size: 769.41 g (27.14 oz-wt.)   Serves: 1

Amount per serving	Food item
10 oz-wt	Cabbage and Celery Soup
4 oz-wt	Kasha with Mushrooms
4 oz-wt	Chicken Breast-Boneless-Roasted
4 oz-wt	Buttercup Squash with Onions and Tarragon

Chicken Dinner *continued*

Amount per serving continued   *Food item* continued

1 cup	Tossed Green Salad
1 tsp	Olive Oil
¹/₂ tsp	Fresh Lemon Juice

Nutrients per serving

Calories	475.99
Protein	42.94 g
Carbohydrates	45.20 g
Dietary fiber	10.32 g
Percent Calories from fat	28%
Fat—Total	15.40 g
Saturated fat	3.74 g
Vitamin A	489.96 RE
Vitamin C	32.87 mg
Percent calories from carbohydrates	37%

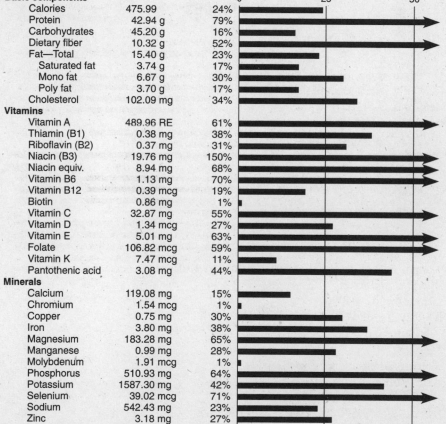

Nutrient	Value	Percent of daily nutrient allowance per serving
Basic components		
Calories	475.99	24%
Protein	42.94 g	79%
Carbohydrates	45.20 g	16%
Dietary fiber	10.32 g	52%
Fat—Total	15.40 g	23%
Saturated fat	3.74 g	17%
Mono fat	6.67 g	30%
Poly fat	3.70 g	17%
Cholesterol	102.09 mg	34%
Vitamins		
Vitamin A	489.96 RE	61%
Thiamin (B1)	0.38 mg	38%
Riboflavin (B2)	0.37 mg	31%
Niacin (B3)	19.76 mg	150%
Niacin equiv.	8.94 mg	68%
Vitamin B6	1.13 mg	70%
Vitamin B12	0.39 mcg	19%
Biotin	0.86 mg	1%
Vitamin C	32.87 mg	55%
Vitamin D	1.34 mcg	27%
Vitamin E	5.01 mg	63%
Folate	106.82 mcg	59%
Vitamin K	7.47 mcg	11%
Pantothenic acid	3.08 mg	44%
Minerals		
Calcium	119.08 mg	15%
Chromium	1.54 mcg	1%
Copper	0.75 mg	30%
Iron	3.80 mg	38%
Magnesium	183.28 mg	65%
Manganese	0.99 mg	28%
Molybdenum	1.91 mcg	1%
Phosphorus	510.93 mg	64%
Potassium	1587.30 mg	42%
Selenium	39.02 mcg	71%
Sodium	542.43 mg	23%
Zinc	3.18 mg	27%

RESOURCES AND REFERENCES

RESOURCES

Annemarie Colbin, C.H.E.S.
The Natural Gourmet Cookery School
The Natural Gourmet Institute for Food and Health
48 West 21st Street, 2nd floor
New York, NY 10010
Tel.: (212) 645-5170

*The Institute offers classes in natural foods cooking, lectures on natural healing top-
ics, and Friday Night Dinners. The School offers a chef's training program in natural
foods cooking, and is licensed by the New York State Education Department. Ms. Colbin can be reached for lectures, seminars, and lifestyle and wellness consultations.*

Organizations

Women to Women—Christiane Northrup, M.D.
One Pleasant Street
Yarmouth, ME 04096
Tel.: (207) 846-6163

A clinic that treats women holistically.

Women's International Pharmacy
5708 Monona Drive
Madison, WI 53716
Tel.: (800) 279-5708 and (608) 221-7800; fax: (608) 221-7819

Natural hormone therapy by prescription only.

The Energy Bank—Nina Merer, C.H.E.S., M.Th., President
157 West 76th Street
New York, NY 10023
Tel.: (212) 877-5060
   Stress and energy management, corporate seminars, and private sessions.

Mountain Ark Trading Company
120 South East Avenue
Fayetteville, AR 72701
Tel.: (800) 643-8909
   Mail order natural foods store, including grains, beans, sea vegetables, cookware, and much more. Call for catalog.

Maine Seaweed Company
P.O. Box 57
Steuben, ME 04680
Tel.: (207) 546-2875
   Local sea vegetables obtained with ecologically sound harvesting techniques from the Maine coast. Call for catalog.

National Women's Health Network
514 10th Street, NW, Suite 400
Washington, DC 20004
Tel.: (202) 628-7814; fax: (202) 347-1168
   Activist-oriented, committed organization supporting the health of women. Does not follow the mainstream, but collects and disseminates information from many original sources. Publishers of the newsletter The Network News, *an excellent, clear-headed publication dealing with women's health issues.*

Newsletters

What Doctors Don't Tell You
Lynne McTaggart, ed.
4 Wallace Road
London N1 2PG, Great Britain

Women's Health Letter
Kerry Bodner, ed.
P.O. Box 467939
Atlanta, GA 31146-7939
Tel.: 800-728-2288 or 770-399-5617

Dr. Christiane Northrup's
Health Wisdom for Women—Intelligent,
Sensitive Solutions to Your Health Concerns
Phillips Publishing Inc.
7811 Montrose Road
Potomac, MD 20854
E-mail: cnorthrup@phillips.com

REFERENCES

Books

Appleton, Nancy, Ph.D., *Healthy Bones: What You Should Know About Osteoporosis.* Avery Publishing Group, Garden City, NY: 1991.

Black, Dean, Ph.D., *Health at the Crossroads.* Tapestry Press, Springville, UT: 1988.

Colbin, A., *Food and Healing.* Ballantine Books, NY: 1996.

Crayhon, Robert, *Robert Crayhon's Nutrition Made Simple.* M. Evans and Company, NY: 1994.

Dunne, Lavon J., *Nutrition Almanac.* McGraw-Hill Publishers, NY.

Erasmus, Udo, *Fats that Heal, Fats that Kill.* Alive Books, Burnaby, BC, Canada: 1993.

Gaby, Alan R., M.D., *Preventing and Reversing Osteoporosis—What You Can Do About Bone Loss.* Prima Publishing, Rocklin, CA: 1994.

Gittleman, Ann Louise, M.S., C.N.S., *Supernutrition for Menopause.* Pocket Books, NY: 1993.

Goulder, Lois; Lutwak, Leo, M.D., Ph.D., *The Strong Bones Diet: The High Calcium Low Calorie Way to Prevent Osteoporosis.* Triad Publishing Co., Gainesville, FL: 1988.

Hands, Elizabeth S. *The Food Finder: Food Sources of Vitamins and Minerals* (companion book to "The Food Processor II" Diet Analysis Software). ESHA Research, Salem, Oregon: 1990.

Jacobowitz, Ruth S., *150 Most-Asked Questions About Osteoporosis: What Women Really Want to Know.* Hearst Books, NY: 1993.

Lark, Susan M., M.D., *The Menopause Self Help Book: A Woman's Guide to Feeling Wonderful for the Second Half of Her Life.* Celestial Arts, Berkeley, CA: 1992.

Myss, Caroline, *Anatomy of the Spirit: The Seven Stages of Power and Healing.* Harmony Books, NY: 1996.

Northrup, Christiane, M.D., *Women's Bodies, Women's Wisdom: Creating Physical and Emotional Health and Healing.* Bantam Books, NY: 1994.

Ohsawa, George, *Essential Ohsawa: From Food to Health, Happiness to Freedom,* Carl Ferré, ed. Avery Publishing Group, Garden City, NY: 1994.

Ojeda, Linda, Ph.D., *Menopause Without Medicine.* Hunter House, Alameda, CA: 1995.

Price, Weston, D.D.S., *Nutrition and Physical Degeneration* (50th Anniversary Edition). Keats Publishing, New Canaan, CT: 1989.

Shils, Maurice E.; Olson, James A.; Shike, Moshe, *Modern Nutrition in Health and Disease* (8th edition). Lea & Febiger, PA: 1994.

Stitt, Paul A., *Beating the Food Giants.* Natural Press, Manitowoc, WI.

Visser, Margaret, *Much Depends on Dinner: The Extraordinary History and Mythology, Allure and Obsessions, Perils and Taboos of an Ordinary Meal.* Grove Press, NY: 1986.

Watson, George, Ph.D., *Nutrition and Your Mind.* Harper & Row, NY: 1972.

Winter, Ruth, M.S., *A Consumer's Guide to Medicines in Food.* Crown Trade Paperbacks, NY: 1995.

Articles and papers

Abbott, L; Nadler, J; Rude, R.K., "Magnesium deficiency in alcoholism: possible contribution to osteoporosis and cardiovascular disease in alcoholism." *Alcohol Clin Esp Res* 1994; **18**(5):1076–1082.

Antonios, T.F.; MacGregor, G.A., "Salt intake: potential deleterious effects excluding blood pressure." *J Hum Hypertens* 1995; **9**(6):511–515.

Beall, D.P.; Scofield, R.H., "Milk-alkali syndrome associated with calcium carbonate consumption. Report of seven patients with parathyroid hormone levels and an estimate of prevalence among patients hospitalized with hypercalcemia." *Medicine* 1995; **74**(2):89–96.

Brody, Jane, "The war on brittle bones must start early in life." The *New York Times,* June 15, 1994. Information packet on "Osteoporosis," from the National Women's Health Network, Washington, DC.

Brody, Jane, "When bones are weakening, several treatments can help save them." The *New York Times,* September 30, 1997.

Brown, Susan, E., "Osteoporosis: sorting fact from fallacy." *The Network News,* July/August 1988, National Women's Health Network, Washington, DC.

Buckwalter J.A.; Glimcher M.J.; Cooper R.R.; Recker R., "Bone Biology I: structure, blood supply, cells, matrix, and mineralization." *Bone.Biology and Tumors* Inst. Course Lecture 1996; 45: 371–386.

Carmichael, K.A.; Fallon, M.D.; Dalinka, M.; Kaplan, F.S.; Axel, L.; Haddad, J.G., "Osteomalacia and osteitis fibrosa in a man ingesting aluminum hydroxide antacid." *American Journal of Medicine* 1984; **76**(6):1137–1143.

Cauley, J.A.; Lucas, F.L.; Kuller, L.H.; Vogt, M.T.; Browner, W.S.; Cummings, S.R., "Bone mineral density and risk of breast cancer in older women: the study of osteoporotic fractures." *JAMA* 1996; **276**(17):1404–1408.

Chang, J.C.; Edelstein, S.L., "Coffee-associated osteoporosis offset by daily milk consumption." *JAMA* 1994; **27**(4):280–283.

Colbin, A., "The calcium question." *Free Spirit Magazine,* June 1987.

Colditz, G.A.; Stampfer, M.J.; Rosner, B.; Speizer, F.E.; Willett, W.C., "Caffeine, moderate alcohol intake, and risk of fractures of the hip and forearm in middle aged women." Channing Laboratory, Department of Medicine, Brigham and Women's Hospital, Boston.

Cooper, C.; Atkinson, E.J.; Wahner, H.W.; O'Fallon, W.M.; et al., "Is caffeine consumption a risk factor for osteoporosis?" *J Bone Miner Res* 1992; **7** (4): 465–471.

Cotrozzi, G.; Relli, P., "Osteoporosis. Current advances in etiopathogenesis, diagnosis, and therapy. I." *Clin Ter* 1994; **144**(3):251–263.

Cowan, T., M.D., "Nutrition and behavior." *Health Journal* 1997; **21**(1):10–11.

Cumming, R.G.; Cummings, S.R.; Nevitt, M.C.; Scott, J.; Ensrud, K.E.; Vogt, T.M.; Fox, K., "Calcium intake and fracture risk: results from the study of osteoporotic fractures." *American Journal of Epidemiology* 1997; **145** (10): 926–934.

Crilly, R.G.; Delaquierriere-Richardson, L., "Current bone mass and body weight changes in alcoholic males." *Calcif Tissue Int* 1990; **46**(3):169–172.

Daly, E.; Vessey, M.P.; Hawkins, M.M.; Carson, J.L.; Gough, P.; Marsh, S., "Risk of venous thromboembolism in users of hormone replacement therapy." *Lancet* 1996; **348**(9033):977–980.

Dawson-Hughes, B., M.D., "Osteoporosis and aging: gastrointestinal aspects." *Journal of the American College of Nutrition* 1986; **5**:393–398.

Devine, A.; Criddle, R.A.; Dick, I.M.; Kerr, D.A.; Prince, R.L., "A longitudinal study of the effect of sodium and calcium intakes on regional bone density in postmenopausal women." *Am J Clin Nutri* 1995; **62**(4):740–745.

Di Costanzo, D., "Fruit smoothie." *Self* magazine, July 1995, p. 133.

Evans, W.J., "Effects of exercise on body composition and functional capacity of the elderly." *J Geront A Biol Schi Med Sci* 1995; **50**:147–150.

Fallon, S., Enig, M.G., Ph.D., "Out of Africa: what Dr. Price and Dr. Burkitt discovered in their studies of sub-Saharan tribes." *Health Journal* 1997; **21** (1):1–5.

Fallon, S., Enig, M.G., Ph.D., "Dem Bones—do high protein diets cause bone loss?" *Health Journal,* 1996; **20**(2).

Felson, D.T.; Zhang, Y.; et al., "Alcohol intake and bone mineral density in elderly men and women." *Am J Epidemiol* 1995; **142**(5):485–492.

Feskanich, D.; Willett, W.C.; Stampfer, M.J.; Colditz, G.A., "Milk, dietary calcium, and bone fracture risk in women: a 12-year prospective study." *American Journal of Public Health* 1997; **87**(6):992–997.

Franklin, D., "The big lift." *Health,* March/April 1996.

Fuchs, N.K., Ph.D., "Calcium controversy." In *Women's Health Letter*—the *Monthly Review of Women's Health Issues,* March 1993.

Gilbert, S., "Weight loss after 50 can be hazardous for women." *New York Times,* June 4, 1996.

Graf, E.; Eaton, J.W. "Dietary phytate and calcium bioavailability." In *Nutritional Bioavailability of Calcium,* Constance Kies, ed. Based on a symposium at the 187th meeting of the American Chemical Society, St. Louis, MO, April 8–13, 1984. American Chemical Society, Washington, DC: 1985.

Health News, "More drugs, more problems." September 17, 1996.

Hillier, S.; Inskip, H.; Coggon, D.; Cooper, C., "Water fluoridation and osteoporotic fracture." *Community Dental Health* 1996; **13**(Suppl 2):S63–S68.

Jobst K.; and Nagy J., "Can aluminum-containing antacid produce dementia?" *Nephron* 1995; **71**(4):473.

Josse, R.G., "Prevention and management of osteoporosis: consensus statements from the Scientific Advisory Board of the Osteoporosis Society of Canada. 3. Effects of ovarian hormone therapy on skeletal and extraskeletal tissues in women." *Can Med Assoc Journal,* 1996; **155**(7):929–934.

Kanis, J.A., "Estrogens, the menopause, and osteoporosis." *Bone,* 1996; **19**: 185S–190S.

Karagas, M.R.; Baron, J.A.; Jacobsen, S.J., "Patterns of fracture among the United States elderly: geographic and fluoride effects." *Annals of Epidemiology* 1996; **6**(3):209–216.

Kleerekoper, M., "Fluoride and the skeleton." *Critical Reviews in Clinical Laboratory Sciences* 1996; **33**(2):139–161.

Klesges, R.C.; Ward, K.D.; Shelton, M.L.; et al., "Changes in bone mineral content in male athletes. Mechanisms of action and intervention effects." *JAMA* 1996; **276**(3):226–230.

Legrand, E.; Le Levier, F.; Chappard, D.; Audran, M., "Male osteoporosis." *Rev Prat* 1994; **44**(12):1563–1568.

Liberman, U.A., et al., "Effect of oral alendronate on bone mineral density and the incidence of fractures in postmenopausal osteoporosis." *The New England Journal of Medicine,* 1995; **333**(22):1437–1443.

Lichtman, R., "Perimenopausal and postmenopausal hormone replacement therapy. Part 1. An update of the literature on benefits and risks." *Journal of Nurse-Midwifery* 1966; **41**(3):228–229.

Massey, L.K.; Whiting, S.J., "Caffeine, urinary calcium, calcium metabolism and bone." *J Nutr* 1993; **123**(9):1611–1614.

May, H.; Reader, R.; Murphy, S.; Khaw, K.T., "Self-reported tooth loss and bone mineral density in older men and women." *Age and Aging* 1995; **24** (3):217–221.

Meyer, H.E.; Pederson, J.I.; Loken, E.B.; Tverdal, A., "Dietary factors and the incidence of hip fracture in middle-aged Norwegians. A prospective study." *Am J Epidemiology* 1997; **145**(2):117–223.

Mohammad, A.R.; Brunsvold, M.; Bauer, R., "The strength of association between systemic postmenopausal osteoporosis and periodontal disease." *Int J Prosthodont* 1996; **9**(5):479–483.

Montague, P., "Genetic engineering error." *Rachel's Environmental Health Weekly*

549, June 5, 1997. (Environmental Research Foundation, P.O. Box 5036, Annapolis, MD 21403.)

Muldowney, W.P.; Mazbar, S.A., "Rolaids–yogurt syndrome: a 1990's version of milk-alkali syndrome." *American Journal of Kidney Diseases* 1996; **27** (2):270–272.

New York Times, "Risks seen in using certain sleeping aids." December 19, 1989.

New York Times, "Exercise aids older women." April 28, 1997.

Nidecker, A., "Alendronate also prevents hip and wrist fractures." *Internal Medicine News,* February 1, 1997, p. 28.

Niewoehner, C.B., "Osteoporosis in men. Is it more common than we think?" *Postgrad Med* 1993; (**8**):59–60, 63–70.

Nnakwe, N.; Ries, C., "Mouse bone composition and breaking strength: effects of varying calcium and phosphorus content in animal or plant protein diets." In *Nutritional Bioavailability of Calcium*, Constance Kies, ed. Based on a symposium at the 187th meeting of the American Chemical Society, St. Louis, MO, April 8–13, 1984. American Chemical Society, Washington, DC: 1985.

Northrup, C., "Ensure a firm health foundation: diet and nutrition for your bones." *Health Wisdom for Women,* March 1998, Vol. 5, No. 3, pp. 1–3.

Nutrition Action Health Letter, "Vitamin D deficiency: the silent epidemic." Center for Science in the Public Interest, 1997; **24**(8).

Olschewski, P.; Nordmeyer, J.P.; Scholten, T., "The milk-alkali syndrome—a rare differential diagnosis for hypercalcemia." *Deutsche Medizinische Wochenschrift* 1996; **121**(33):1015–1018.

Ott, S.M. "Bone mass measurements: reasons to be cautious—Bone mass and strength not necessarily correlated." [letter] *British Medical Journal,* 1994; **308**, 931–932.

Ott, S.M., "Clinical effects of bisphosphonates in involutional osteoporosis." *Journal of Bone and Mineral Research* 1993; **8** Suppl 2:S597–S606.

Ott, S.M., "When bone mass fails to predict bone failure." *Calcified Tissue International* 1993; **53** Suppl 1:S7–S13.

Pearson, D.; McTaggart, L., "Osteoporosis: a load of old bones." *What Doctors Don't Tell You,* 1996; **6**(12).

Pritchard, J.E.; Nowson, C.A.; Wark, J.D., "Bone loss accompanying diet-induced or exercise-induced weight loss: a randomised controlled study." *International Journal of Obesity and Related Metabolic Disorders* 1996; **20** (6):513–520.

Ravn, S.H.; Rosenberg, J.; Bostofte, E., "Postmenopausal hormone replacement therapy—clinical implications." *Eur. J. Obst. Reprod. Biol.* 1994; **53** (2): 81–93.

Ray, W.A.; Griffin, M.R.; Downey, W., "Benzodiazepines of long and short elimination half-life and the risk of hip fracture." *JAMA* 1989; **262** (23): 3303–3307.

Runowicz, C., "Hormone therapy: when and for how long?" *HealthNews,* March 25, 1997.

Saltman; P.D., Strause, L.G., "The role of trace minerals in osteoporosis." *Journal of the Americal College of Nutrition* 1993; **12**(4):384–389.

Shaw, C.K., "An epidemiologic study of osteoporosis in Taiwan." *Annals of Epidemiology* 1993; **3**:264–271.

Silverman, K.; Evans, S.M.; Strain, E.C.; Griffiths, R.R., "Withdrawal syndrome after the double blind cessation of caffeine consumption." *N Engl J Med* 1992; **327**:1109–1114.

Skotowski, M.C.; Hunt, R.J.; Levy, S.M., "Risk factors for dental fluorosis in pediatric dental patients." *Journal of Public Health Dentistry* 1995; **55** (3): 154–159.

Spencer, H.; Kramer, L., "Osteoporosis, calcium requirement, and factors causing calcium loss." *Clin Geriatr Med* 1987 May; **3**:389–402—"Factors contributing to osteoporosis." *Journal of Nutrition* 1986; **116**:316–319—Further studies of the effect of a high protein diet as meat on calcium metabolism." *Am J Clin Nutr* 1983 June; **37**:924–929.

The Network News, "ERT: if it's so great, why aren't we all on it? Or, from noncompliance to new understanding." Published by the National Women's Health Network. January/February 1997.

Thomas, W.C. Jr., "Exercise, age, and the bones," *Southern Medical Journal,* 1994; **87**(4):S23–S25.

Tohyama, E., "Relationship between fluoride concentration in drinking water and mortality rate from uterine cancer in Okinawa prefecture, Japan." *Journal of Epidemiology* 1996 Dec; **6**(4):184–81.

Tsukahara, J.; Toda, A.; Goto, J.; Ezawa, W., "Cross-sectional and longitudinal studies on the effect of water exercise in controlling bone loss in Japanese postmenopausal women." *Journal of Nutritional Science and Vitaminology* (Tokyo) 1994; **40**(1):37–47.

Tufts University *Health & Nutrition Letter,* "Like to walk? Put away your walking shoes." 1997; **15**(2):1.

Watkins, T.R.; Pandya, K., Mickelsen, O., "Urinary acid and calcium excretion: effect of soy vs meat in human diets." In *Nutritional Bioavailability of Calcium,* Constance Kies, ed. Based on a symposium at the 187th meeting of the American Chemical Society, St. Louis, MO, April 8–13, 1984. American Chemical Society, Washington, DC: 1985.

Williams, S., "Caffeine in your decaf?" *Self* magazine, March 1996.

Winthrow, C.D., "The ketogenic diet: mechanism of anticonvulsant action." In *Antiepileptic Drugs: Mechanisms of Action,* G.H. Glaser, J.K. Penry, and D.M. Woodbury, eds. Raven Press, NY.

Wilford, J.N., "Volcano preserved corn, chilies, and house mice." *New York Times,* April 8, 1997.

What Doctors Don't Tell You, "HRT: dense bones lead to cancer." January 1997.

INDEXES

RECIPE INDEX

INDEX

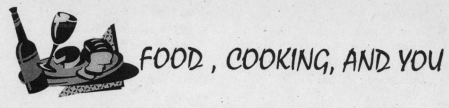

FOOD , COOKING, AND YOU

FROM PENGUIN PUTNAM INC.

☐**THE ALL-IN-ONE DIABETIC COOKBOOK**
by P.J. Palumbo, M.D. and Joyce Daly Margie
0-452-26467-7/$13.95

☐**THE CARBOHYDRATE ADDICT'S LIFESPAN PROGRAM**
by Dr. Richard Heller and Dr. Rachael Heller
0-452-27838-4/$14.95

☐**HIGH-FLAVOR, LOW-FAT VEGETARIAN COOKING**
by Steven Raichlen
0-14-024124-8/$18.95

☐**THE SOY GOURMET** by Robin Robertson
0-452-27922-4/$11.95

Prices slightly higher in Canada.